Biology of
Acetabularia

Proceedings of the First International Symposium on
Acetabularia organized jointly by the Université Libre
de Bruxelles, Brussels (Belgium) and the Centre d'Etude
de l'Energie Nucléaire, Mol (Belgium), under the aus-
pices of the European Communities (EURATOM), held in
Brussels and in Mol, June 18-20, 1969.

Biology of
Acetabularia

Edited by

Jean Brachet

Laboratoire de Morphologie Animale
Faculté des Sciences
Université Libre de Bruxelles
Brussels, Belgium

and

Silvano Bonotto

Département de Radiobiologie
Centre d'Etude de l'Energie Nucléaire
Mol, Belgium

Academic Press • New York • London • 1970

ACADEMIC PRESS, INC.
111 Fifth Avenue, New York, New York 10003

United Kingdom Edition published by
ACADEMIC PRESS, INC. (LONDON) LTD.
Berkeley Square House, London W1X 6BA

LIBRARY OF CONGRESS CATALOG CARD NUMBER: 74-117084

PRINTED IN THE UNITED STATES OF AMERICA

PARTICIPANTS

Johannes Anders, Institut für Biologie der Universität Tübingen, Germany

Klaus Apel, Max-Planck-Institut für Zellbiologie, Wilhelmshaven, Germany

Cyrille Baes, Département de Radiobiologie, Centre d'Etude de l'Energie Nucléaire, Mol, Belgium

Wilfried Baeyens, Département de Radiobiologie, Centre d'Etude de l'Energie Nucléaire, Mol, Belgium

Eliane Baltus, Laboratoire de Morphologie Animale, Faculté des Sciences, Université Libre de Bruxelles, Brussels, Belgium

Lucile Baugnet-Mahieu, Département de Radiobiologie, Centre d'Etude de l'Energie Nucléaire, Mol, Belgium

Sigrid Berger, Max-Planck-Institut für Zellbiologie, Wilhelmshaven, Germany

Denise Bernaert, Laboratoire de Chimie Biologique, Faculté des Sciences, Université Libre de Bruxelles, Brussels, Belgium

Albert Jacques Bertinchamps, EURATOM, Service de Biologie, Brussels, Belgium

Kurt Beth, Stazione Zoologica, Napoli, Italy

Monique Boloukhère, Laboratoire de Morphologie Animale, Faculté des Sciences, Université Libre de Bruxelles, Brussels, Belgium

Eliane Bonnijns-Van Gelder, Département de Radiobiologie, Centre d'Etude de l'Energie Nucléaire, Mol, Belgium

Silvano Bonotto, Département de Radiobiologie, Centre d'Etude de l'Energie Nucléaire, Mol, Belgium

Jean Brachet, Laboratoire de Morphologie Animale, Faculté des Sciences, Université Libre de Bruxelles, Brussels, Belgium

Ernst P.O. Brändle, Institut für Biologie der Universität Tübingen, Germany

Raymond André Bronchart, Institut de Botanique, Université de Liège, Belgium

Marianne Cape, Laboratoire de Morphologie Animale, Faculté des Sciences, Université Libre de Bruxelles, Brussels, Belgium

Hubert Chantrenne, Laboratoire de Chimie Biologique, Faculté des Sciences, Université Libre de Bruxelles, Brussels, Belgium

Pol Charles, Département de Radiobiologie, Centre d'Etude de l'Energie Nucléaire, Mol, Belgium

Heins Clauss, Pflanzenphysiologisches Institut der Freien Universität Berlin, Berlin-Dahlem, Germany

Claude Cocriamont, Laboratoire de Chimie Biologique, Faculté des Sciences, Université Libre de Bruxelles, Brussels, Belgium

Paul Coucke, Laboratorium voor Fysiologische Chemie, Fakulteit der Geneeskunde, Rijksuniversiteit-Gent, Gent, Belgium

J. C. W. Crawley, Medical Research Council, Clinical Research Centre, Radio-isotopes Division, Guy's Hospital Medical School, London, England

Maud Decroly, Laboratoire de Morphologie Animale, Faculté des Sciences, Université Libre de Bruxelles, Brussels, Belgium

Françoise de Vitry, Laboratoire de Génétique Cellulaire, Institut Pasteur, Paris, France

Walter L. Dillard, Max-Planck-Institut für Zellbiologie, Wilhelmshaven, Germany

Esther Dujardin, Centre de Recherche de Gorsem, Sint-Truiden, Belgium

Maurice Errera, Laboratoire de Biophysique et Radiobiologie, Faculté des Sciences, Université Libre de Bruxelles, Brussels, Belgium

Eugène Fagniart, Département de Radiobiologie, Centre d'Etude de l'Energie Nucléaire, Mol, Belgium

Nora Fautrez-Firlefyn, Laboratory of Anatomy, University of Gent, Belgium

Adrienne Ficq, Laboratoire de Morphologie Animale, Faculté des Sciences, Université Libre de Bruxelles, Brussels, Belgium

André Goffeau, EURATOM, Service de Biologie, and Laboratoire de Morphologie Animale, Université Libre de Bruxelles, Brussels, Belgium

PARTICIPANTS

Beverley R. Green, Department of Botany, University of British Columbia, Vancouver, Canada

Gerd Ernst Grieninger, Institut für Biologie der Universität Tübingen, Germany

Jacqueline Guermant, Laboratoire de Morphologie Animale, Faculté des Sciences, Université Libre de Bruxelles, Brussels, Belgium

Françoise-Andrée Hanocq, Laboratoire de Morphologie Animale, Faculté des Sciences, Université Libre de Bruxelles, Brussels, Belgium

Jacqueline Hanocq-Quertier, Laboratoire de Morphologie Animale, Faculté des Sciences, Université Libre de Bruxelles, Brussels, Belgium

Viviane Heilporn, Laboratoire de Morphologie Animale, Faculté des Sciences, Université Libre de Bruxelles, Brussels, Belgium

Frank Hellmann, Pflanzenphysiologisches Institut der Freien Universität Berlin, Berlin-Dahlem, Germany

Jacques Homès, Laboratoire de Morphologie Végétale, Université Libre de Bruxelles, Brussels, Belgium

Nicole Hulin, Laboratoire de Morphologie Animale, Faculté des Sciences, Université Libre de Bruxelles, Brussels, Belgium

Michel Janowski, Laboratoire de Morphologie Animale, Faculté des Sciences, Université Libre de Bruxelles, Brussels, Belgium

René Kirchmann, Département de Radiobiologie, Centre d'Etude de l'Energie Nucléaire, Mol, Belgium

Erika Kos, Laboratory of Cellular Biochemistry, Institute "Ruđjer Bošković," Zagreb, Yugoslavia

Luc Lateur, Laboratoire de Morphologie Animale, Faculté des Sciences, Université Libre de Bruxelles, Brussels, Belgium

Ruth Laub - Kupersztejn, Laboratoire de Morphologie Animale, Faculté des Sciences, Université Libre de Bruxelles, Brussels, Belgium

François E.E. Ledoux, Institut de Botanique, Université de Liège, Belgium

Andrée Lievens, Laboratoire de Morphologie Animale, Faculté des Sciences, Université Libre de Bruxelles, Brussels, Belgium

Sylvie Limbosch, Laboratoire de Morphologie Animale, Faculté des Sciences, Université Libre de Bruxelles, Brussels, Belgium

Gerno Linden, Departement de Radiobiologie, Centre d'Etude de l'Energie Nucléaire, Mol, Belgium

Angela Lüttke, Pflanzenphysiologisches Institut der Freien Universität Berlin, Berlin-Dahlem, Germany

Ingrid Maass, Pflanzenphysiologisches Institut der Freien Universität Berlin, Berlin-Dahlem, Germany

Jean-René Maisin, Département de Radiobiologie, Centre d'Etude de l'Energie Nucléaire, Mol, Belgium

Pamela Malpoix, Laboratoire de Morphologie Animale, Faculté des Sciences, Université Libre de Bruxelles, Brussels, Belgium

Paul Manil, Faculté des Sciences Agronomiques de l'Etat, Gembloux, Belgium

Marc Mareel, Laboratory of Radiotherapy, Clinical Academy, University of Gent, Belgium

Maurice Michel, Laboratoire de Morphologie Végétale, Université Libre de Bruxelles, Brussels, Belgium

Simone Puiseux-Dao, Laboratoire de Biologie Cellulaire Végétale, Faculté des Sciences, Université de Paris, France

Hans Jobst Rahmsdorf, Max-Planck-Institut für Zellbiologie, Wilhelmshaven, Germany

Aimée-Marguerite Reuter, Département de Radiobiologie, Centre d'Etude de l'Energie Nucléaire, Mol, Belgium

Wolfgang Reuter, Max-Planck-Institut für Zellbiologie, Wilhelmshaven, Germany

Gerhard Richter, Institut für Botanik, Technische Universität Hannover, Germany

Frank Roels, Laboratory of Human Anatomy, University of Gent, Belgium

Marie-Paul Roels-De Schrijver, Laboratory of Physiology, Veterinary Faculty, University of Gent, Belgium

Ursula Schael, Max-Planck-Institut für Zellbiologie, Wilhelmshaven, Germany

Jozef Schell, Laboratorium voor Genetica, Fakulteit der Wetenschappen, Rijksuniversiteit-Gent, Gent, Belgium

Angèle Schram, Laboratoire de Morphologie Animale, Faculté des Sciences, Université Libre de Bruxelles, Brussels, Belgium

Hans-Georg Schweiger, Max-Planck-Institut für Zellbiologie, Wilhelmshaven, Germany

André A. Sels, Laboratoire de Chimie Biologique, Faculté des Sciences, Université Libre de Bruxelles, Brussels, Belgium

Jean Semal, Laboratoire de Pathologie Végétale, Faculté des Sciences Agronomiques de l'Etat, Gembloux, Belgium

Swetlana Semenoff, Pflanzenphysiologische Institut der Freien Universität Berlin, Berlin-Dahlem, Germany

David C. Shephard, Department of Anatomy, Case Western Reserve University, Cleveland, Ohio

Cyrille H. V. Sironval, Laboratoire de Photobiologie, Université de Liège, Belgium

Nicole Six, Laboratoire de Morphologie Animale, Faculté des Sciences, Université Libre de Bruxelles, Brussels, Belgium

Maurice Steinert, Laboratoire de Morphologie Animale, Faculté des Sciences, Université Libre de Bruxelles, Brussels, Belgium

Renée Tencer, Laboratoire de Morphologie Animale, Faculté des Sciences, Université Libre de Bruxelles, Brussels, Belgium

Jacqueline Thirion, Laboratoire de Morphologie Animale, Faculté des Sciences, Université Libre de Bruxelles, Brussels, Belgium

René Thomas, Laboratoire de Génétique, Faculté des Sciences, Université Libre de Bruxelles, Brussels, Belgium

Oscar Van der Borght, Département de Radiobiologie, Centre d'Etude de l'Energie Nucléaire, Mol, Belgium

Thérèse Vanden Driessche, Laboratoire de Morphologie Animale, Faculté des Sciences, Université Libre de Bruxelles, Brussels, Belgium

Paulette Van Gansen, Laboratoire de Morphologie Animale, Faculté des Sciences, Université Libre de Bruxelles, Brussels, Belgium

Patrick Van Oostveldt, Laboratorium voor Fysiologische Chemie, Fakulteit der Geneeskunde, Rijksuniversiteit-Gent, Gent, Belgium

PARTICIPANTS

Sylvain Van Puymbroeck, Département de Radiobiologie, Centre d'Etude de l'Energie Nucléaire, Mol, Belgium

Jacques Verhulst, Laboratoire de Morphologie Animale, Faculté des Sciences, Université Libre de Bruxelles, Brussels, Belgium

Günther Werz, Max-Planck-Institut für Zellbiologie, Wilhelmshaven, Germany

Klaus Zetsche, Institut für Biologie der Universität Tübingen, Germany

INTRODUCTION

Acetabularia would never have become a highly respectable material and would not have received the honors of an international symposium without the pioneer work of J. Hämmerling in the 1930–1940 period. He first demonstrated that this giant alga has a single nucleus and is therefore a unicellular organism. He then showed that the alga can easily be cut into two halves (nucleate and anucleate) and that, surprisingly, the anucleate fragments undergo a complex morphogenesis (cap formation). This famous experiment demonstrated not only that the cytoplasm can survive for weeks and even months in the absence of the nucleus, but also that it is capable of regenerating, by itself, complicated morphological structures. More delicate experiments of Hämmerling involved interspecific grafts, for instance, a combination between an anucleate half of one species and a nucleate fragment of another. These experiments led to the important conclusion that the nucleus, in *Acetabularia,* produces species-specific *morphogenetic substances* which can retain their activity in the absence of the nucleus for several weeks.

Some twenty years went by, however, before *Acetabularia* became an object of interest for biochemists. It was found, in my laboratory, around 1955, that anucleate fragments of *Acetabularia* can synthesize proteins, including specific enzymes. Since it was already well known that the synthesis of specific proteins is under genetic control, a paradoxical situation arose: How could such a synthesis occur when the genes which should direct the synthesis of the specific enzymes in *Acetabularia* have been taken away by surgical removal of the nucleus? The explanation that I proposed, shortly before the discovery of the messenger ribonucleic acids (mRNA's), was that the information present in the genes (nuclear DNA) must be carried to the cytoplasm in the form of stable molecules of RNA. Speaking in terms of modern molecular biology, this means that mRNA's produced by the nucleus move into the cytoplasm, migrate toward the apex of the stalk (where the cap will form), and retain genetic information for several weeks. This is the hypothesis which remains at the origin of many of the papers which were presented at this Symposium.

But it soon became clear that the presence of chloroplasts in the alga introduces serious complications. It was found that the chloroplasts, in

Acetabularia as elsewhere, contain DNA, RNA, and proteins. Since they can replicate, although at a slower rate, in anucleate as well as in nucleate halves, it was discovered that extensive synthesis of DNA, RNA, and proteins occurs in both kinds of fragments. Further analysis, carried on simultaneously in Wilhelmshaven and in Brussels, has led to the conclusion that while chloroplasts display considerable autonomy toward the nucleus, their independance is not absolute. They require factors originating from the nucleus in order to fully express their potentialities.

The purpose of this Symposium was to exchange ideas and information between the various laboratories which are presently engaged in research on *Acetabularia*. Many problems (DNA synthesis, RNA synthesis, regulation of RNA production and enzyme activity, ultrastructure, photosynthesis, effects of physical factors such as light and gamma-radiations and circadian rhythms) have been thoroughly discussed. There was a general agreement on the main points and some disagreement on minor issues. The book will be useful for all those who work or intend to work on *Acetabularia*. It is sincerely hoped that it will induce more and more workers, in the future, to join the "*Acetabularia* Club." A still greater hope is that *Acetabularia* will find, thanks to this book, the place it deserves in the teaching of general biology and biochemistry, since this alga is one of the most fascinating living objects in the world.

Jean Brachet

CONTENTS

JUNE 18 (RHODE-ST-GENÈSE)
MORNING SESSION
Chairman: Kurt Beth

AFTERNOON SESSION
Chairman: Hubert Chantrenne

CONTENTS

CONTENTS

JUNE 18 (RHODE-ST-GENÈSE)
MORNING SESSION

Chairman: Kurt Beth

REGULATORY PROBLEMS IN ACETABULARIA

Hans-Georg Schweiger

Max-Planck-Institut für Zellbiologie,
Wilhelmshaven, Germany

The organism to whom this symposium is dedicated has been classified by J.V.F. Lamouroux in 1816 (Fig. 1). However, it took more than 100 years that Acetabularia attracted major interest and became a tool in modern cell biology. As early as 1926 Max Hartmann and Joachim Hämmerling started experiments which initially were concerned with the sexuality of Acetabularia. Still before these studies could be finished the objective was changed.

In a preliminary note the very first results on the "Entwicklung und Formbildungsvermögen von Acetabularia mediterranea" were published in "Biologisches Zentralblatt" in 1931 (Hämmerling, 1931). In 1929 Max Hartmann had collected samples of Acetabularia mediterranea nearby Rovigno d'Istria and Hämmerling had succeeded to grow and multiply these cells in the laboratory. One of the more important findings of the paper was that Acetabularia is not only a single cell organism as was already known for decades but that it is also a single nucleus organism and that for most of the time this nucleus is localized in the basal part of the cell, in the rhizoid. Since that time Acetabularia has become a useful tool with which Hämmerling and other people have worked in the Kaiser-Wilhelm-Institut in Berlin-Dahlem, then in Rovigno d'Istria and since 20 years in Wilhelmshaven. More than 1 1/2 decades ago Acetabularia was domesticated in Brussels in the host institute.

It is mainly three problems in which Acetabularia proved to be an excellent tool. Indeed, it is one single

3

problem with three different aspects. The problem is that of differentiation and the three aspects are morphogenesis, temporal organization of the cell and nucleus-cytoplasm-interrelationships.

The regulatory processes of differentiation partially become manifest during growth and morphogenesis (Hämmerling, 1963 ; Schweiger, 1969). The species specific sequence of events in the outgrowth of the zygotes, the formation of stalk and whorls and finally the designing of the cap indicates a special form of temporal organization of the cell. This sort of regulation also includes the synthesis of distinct cell components and enzymes during distinct periods of development. Since all these processes occur in anucleate as in nucleate cells although with lower speed one has to assume that the sequence of events can not be under direct control of the nucleus.

Moreover, still other types of temporal organization have been elucidated in the single cell alga Acetabularia. An especially good example is offered by the circadian periodicity of photosynthetic activity as measured by the oxygen production (Sweeney and Haxo, 1961 ; Schweiger, Wallraff and Schweiger, 1964a ; Vanden Driessche, 1966a,b). The increase of the production of oxygen during daytime and the decreased activity during nighttime can be studied on single cells of Acetabularia (von Klitzing and Schweiger, 1969). These rhythmic oscillations are retained under constant conditions, that means, under constant light. Moreover, the rhythm is not ceased even after the removal of the cell nucleus. It is obvious that the regulation which underlies the rhythmicity is not linked to the nucleus in a direct way.

That the nucleus does have a regulatory function on the photosynthesis rhythm has been shown by experiments in which a cell nucleus was transferred into another cell (Schweiger, Wallraff and Schweiger, 1964b) (Fig. 2). The donor cell had been entrained on a rhythm which was distinguished from that of the acceptor cell by 12 hours. Under the influence of the implanted cell nucleus the rhythm of the acceptor cell was shifted so that after a couple of days the rhythm of the acceptor cell coincided with that of the donor cell. In cross experiments both acceptor cells changed their rhythms. This finding raises

the question how the cell nucleus manages to shift the
rhythm. A rather simple explanation would be that this regulation is performed by a nuclear product which becomes
effective in the cytoplasm and most probably in the chloroplasts. It is suggestive to assume that the nuclear product
is mRNA and that this mRNA codes for enzymes which are involved in the mechanism of photosynthesis. In that case
the shift of the rhythm would be accomplished by qualitative and quantitative changes of the enzyme pattern due to
mRNA directed protein synthesis. This assumption is supported by the fact that RNA synthesis in Acetabularia is also
subjected to a diurnal rhythm (Vanden Driessche and Bonotto,
1969). The involvement of mRNA directed protein synthesis
in the mechanism of circadian rhythmicity is suggested by
results which indicate the nuclear dependency of organelle
enzymes. Besides the rhythmicity of photosynthetic activity
with a rather low frequency other oscillations are known
e.g. for the concentration of ATP and for the activity of
enzymes which exhibit substantial higher frequencies (von
Klitzing and Schweiger, 1969). However, the mechanism of
these oscillations is unknown.

The temporal organization of the cell is closely related to the structural organization, that means, that
membrane systems, compartments and cell organelles should
be involved and, as can be concluded from the experiments
on the circadian rhythm, nucleus-cytoplasm interactions
which most probably are nucleus-plastid interactions play
an important part in this regulation. The nucleus-plastid
interaction is in some way contradictory to the fact that
plastids apparently dispose of features which are considered to be prerequisites for genetic autonomy. Plastids of
Acetabularia have been shown to contain DNA (Gibor and
Izawa, 1963 ; Baltus and Brachet, 1963 ; Green et al.,
1967, Berger and Schweiger, 1969) and to be capable of
synthesizing DNA (Gibor, 1967 ; Berger and Schweiger, 1969),
to contain RNA (Naora, Naora and Brachet, 1960 ; Janowski,
1965 ; Schweiger, 1967) and to be capable of synthesizing
RNA (Schweiger and Bremer, 1961 ; Janowski et al., 1969)
as well as protein (Clauss, 1958, Goffeau and Brachet,1965;
Bonotto et al., 1969). However, it has to be postulated
that the nucleus must play a role in the genetic machinery
of the plastids. At least some of the information which
codes for the structural and functional components of the

5

plastids has to be supplied by the nuclear DNA because the amount of DNA per plastid which has been estimated to be in the range of 10^{-16} g (Gibor and Izawa, 1963 ; Baltus and Brachet, 1963) is not sufficient for this purpose.

Experiments which reveal such a contribution of information by the nucleus have been performed on the enzymes malic dehydrogenase (MDH) (Schweiger, Master and Werz,1967) and lactic dehydrogenase (LDH) (Reuter and Schweiger, 1969). Both enzymes can be separated into isozymes if they are subjected to electrophoresis in polyacrylamide gel. The isozyme patterns of the MDH and of the LDH is highly species specific by the number and the position of the enzyme bands. If nuclei of cells of two different species of Acetabularia are exchanged over cross, the isozyme pattern is changed within about 4 weeks so that the old isozyme pattern disappears and a new one which corresponds to the species of the implanted nucleus is formed (Fig. 3;Fig.4). Obviously, the cell has been transformed under the influence of the implanted nucleus with respect to the MDH and the LDH respectively. This finding agrees well with the fact that an implanted nucleus is capable of directing morphogenesis (Hämmerling, 1963). It is interesting enough to note that after the implantation of the heterologous nucleus the isozyme pattern of the cytoplasm disappears although the isozyme pattern not only is retained after enucleation but also the total activity of MDH is increased. There can be no doubt that the disappearance of the isozyme pattern is due to the implanted nucleus. It is suggestive to assume that in the anucleate cell the mRNA is protected and remains functionally intact, while in the presence of an implanted nucleus the homologous mRNA is displaced from the protected form by newly synthesized heterologous RNA. The protection of mRNA might be effected in the polysomal complex or in an mRNA protein aggregate. Special interest is focussed at the localization. It is known that MDH occurs in the mitochondria (Roodyn, 1967). Besides this localization there is some evidence in favour of the idea that MDH also occurs in chloroplasts (Zelitch and Barber, 1960). In the case of Acetabularia it has been shown by means of a histochemical method and by means of the density gradient centrifugation in an anhydrous system that at least part of the enzyme activity is associated with the chloroplasts. In a similar way the LDH has also been demonstrated to be localized at least partially in the chloroplasts. From the results it can be concluded that at least two organelle enzymes namely the MDH and the LDH are coded by nuclear DNA and, moreover, it is probable that at least part of the enzyme activities of both enzymes is linked to the chloroplasts. That does not mean anything else than nuclear dependence of some of the plastid components or, in other words, that in spite of the genetic autonomy of the chloroplasts some of the components of the plastids are coded by nuclear DNA. One may assume that MDH and LDH are not the only enzymes which occur in the plastids and which are coded by the nucleus. Such an interrelationship between cell nucleus and plastids might help to explain the influence of the nucleus on the circadian rhythm and on other plastid functions like RNA synthesis.

References

E. Baltus and J. Brachet, 1963 : Presence of deoxyribonucleic acid in the chloroplasts of Acetabularia mediterranea. Biochim. Biophys. Acta 76, 490-492.

S. Berger and H.G. Schweiger, 1969 : Synthesis of chloroplast DNA in Acetabularia. Physiol. Chem. and Physics 1, 280-292.

S. Bonotto, A. Goffeau, M. Janowski, T. Vanden Driessche and J. Brachet, 1969 : Effects of various inhibitors of protein synthesis on Acetabularia mediterranea. Biochim. Biophys. Acta 174, 704-712.

H. Clauss, 1958 : Über quantitative Veränderungen der Chloroplasten- und cytoplasmatischen Proteine in kernlosen Teilen von Acetabularia mediterranea. Planta 52, 334-350.

A. Gibor, 1967 : DNA synthesis in chloroplast. In : Biochemistry of chloroplasts (ed. T.W. Goodwin), vol. 2, p. 321-328, New York : Academic Press.

A. Gibor and M. Izawa, 1963 : The DNA content of the chloroplasts of Acetabularia. Proc. Nat. Acad. Sci. 50, 1164-1169.

A. Goffeau and J. Brachet, 1965 : Deoxyribonucleic acid-dependent incorporation of amino acids into the proteins of chloroplasts isolated from anucleate Acetabularia fragments. Biochim. Biophys. Acta 95, 302–313.

B. Green, V. Heilporn, S. Limbosch, M. Boloukhère and J. Brachet, 1967 : The cytoplasmic DNA's of Acetabularia mediterranea. Proc. Nat. Acad. Sci. 58, 1351–1358.

J. Hämmerling, 1931 : Entwicklung und Formbildungsvermögen von Acetabularia mediterranea. Biol. Zentralblatt 51, 633–647.

J. Hämmerling, 1963 : Nucleo-cytoplasmic interactions in Acetabularia and other cells. Ann. Rev. Plant Physiol. 14, 65–92.

M. Janowski, 1965 : Synthèse chloroplastique d'acides nucléiques chez Acetabularia mediterranea. Biochim. Biophys. Acta 103, 399–408.

M. Janowski, S. Bonotto and M. Boloukhère, 1969 : Ribosomes of Acetabularia mediterranea. Biochim. Biophys. Acta 174, 525–535.

L. v. Klitzing and H.G. Schweiger, 1969 : A method for recording the circadian rhythm of the oxygen balance in a single cell of Acetabularia mediterranea. Protoplasma 67, 327–332.

J.V.F. Lamouroux, 1816 : Histoire des Polypiers Coralligenes flexibles (ed. A. Caen).

H. Naora, H. Naora and J. Brachet, 1960 ; Studies on independent synthesis of cytoplasmic ribonucleic acids in Acetabularia mediterranea. J. Gen. Physiol. 43, 1083–1102.

W. Reuter and H.G. Schweiger, 1969 : Kernkontrollierte Lactatdehydrogenase in Acetabularia. Protoplasma (in press).

D.B. Roodyn, 1967 : The Mitochondrion (ed. D.B. Roodyn) p. 103–180, London : Academic Press.

E. Schweiger, H.G. Wallraff and H.G. Schweiger, 1964a :
Über tagesperiodische Schwankungen der Sauerstoff-
bilanz kernhaltiger und kernloser Acetabularia
mediterranea. Z. Naturforsch. 19b, 499-505.

E. Schweiger, H.G. Wallraff and H.G. Schweiger, 1964b :
Endogenous circadian rhythm in cytoplasm of Acetabularia : Influence of the nucleus. Science 146,
658-659.

H.G. Schweiger, 1967 : Regulationsprobleme in der einzelli-
gen Alge Acetabularia. Arzneimittelforsch. 17,
1433-1438.

H.G. Schweiger, 1969 : Cell Biology of Acetabularia. Current Topics in Microbiology and Immunology 50, 1-36.

H.G. Schweiger and H.J. Bremer, 1961 :Cytoplasmatische
RNS-Synthese in kernlosen Acetabularien. Biochim.
Biophys. Acta 51, 50-59.

H.G. Schweiger, R.W.P. Master and G. Werz, 1967 : Nuclear
control of a cytoplasmic enzyme in Acetabularia.
Nature 216, 554-557.

B.M. Sweeney and F.T. Haxo, 1961 : Persistence of a photosynthetic rhythm in enucleated Acetabularia. Science
134, 1361-1363.

T. Vanden Driessche, 1966a : Circadian rhythms in Acetabularia : Photosynthetic capacity and chloroplast
shape. Exp. Cell Res. 42, 18-30.

T. Vanden Driessche, 1966b : The role of the nucleus in
the circadian rhythms of Acetabularia mediterranea.
Biochim. Biophys. Acta 126, 456-470.

T. Vanden Driessche and S. Bonotto, 1969 : The circadian
rhythm in RNA synthesis in Acetabularia mediterranea.
Biochim. Biophys. Acta 179, 58-66.

I. Zelitch and G.A. Barber, 1960 : Oxidative enzymes of
Spinach chloroplasts. Plant Physiol. 35, 626-631.

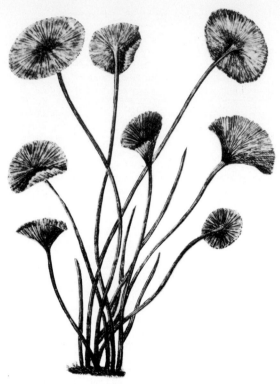

Fig. 1. Acetabularia crenulata (Lamouroux, 1816)

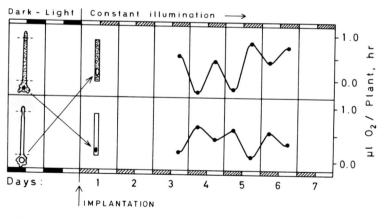

Fig. 2. Influence of the nucleus on the circadian rhythm of photosynthetic activity in Acetabularia mediterranea (Schweiger, Wallraff and Schweiger, 1964b)

10

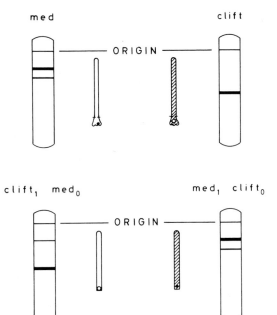

<u>Fig. 3.</u> Influence of the nucleus on the isozyme pattern of MDH (Schweiger, Master and Werz, 1967)

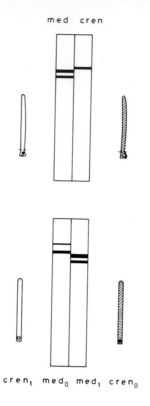

Fig. 4. Influence of the nucleus on the isozyme pattern of LDH (Reuter and Schweiger, 1969)

RNA SYNTHESIS IN ACETABULARIA

Walter L. Dillard

Max-Planck-Institut für Zellbiologie,
Wilhelmshaven, Germany

The comparison of RNA synthesis in nucleate and
enucleated Acetabularia cells has long been held to be one
of the more promising approaches to the problem of charac-
terizing the morphogenetic behavior of this cell in molecular terms. The usefulness of this method has been limited
by several factors which are to a greater or lesser extent
unique to Acetabularia and to the techniques applicable to
its study. Among the more important of these factors are :
(1) the difficulty encountered in consistently preparing
undegraded RNA ; (2) the reaction of Acetabularia to the
trauma associated with the enucleation procedure ; and (3)
the complications introduced by the simultaneous transcription of RNA from several different classes of DNA.

The observation that ribosomal RNA preparations from
Acetabularia are frequently degraded in the presence of substances which have been shown to be effective inhibitors of
Acetabularia ribonucleases in vitro indicates that the ribonucleases exist in close association with or bound to the
ribosomes. Under these conditions the major part of the degradation occurs during homogenization of the cells at a
time before inhibitors can have access to the ribonucleases.
All or most of the difficulties encountered in preparing
undegraded RNA from Acetabularia can be eliminated by modification of the homogenization procedure.

The tendency of RNA preparations from enucleated cells
to be more frequently degraded than preparations from intact
cells apears to be due to a response of Acetabularia to the

trauma of enucleation in which ribosomal RNA is degraded. This trauma-induced degradation is spontaneously reversible. Undegraded RNA can be consistently prepared from enucleated cells if they are allowed to recover for 10 days or more under standard culture conditions.

The kinetics of incorporation of radioactive precursors into the "heavy" and "light" peaks of Acetabularia RNA indicate that these peaks are heterogenous. Recent experimental results support the conclusions of the kinetic studies and have shown that there are small, but consistent differences in the sedimentation behavior of the components comprising the peaks.

AFTERNOON SESSION

Chairman: Hubert Chantrenne

A STABLE RNA SPECIES
IN ACETABULARIA MEDITERRANEA

Michel Janowski[x]

Laboratoire de Morphologie Animale
Université Libre de Bruxelles,
Brussels, Belgium

and

Silvano Bonotto

Département de Radiobiologie
Centre d'Etude de l'Energie Nucléaire,
Mol, Belgium.

Abstract

1. The RNA's of Acetabularia mediterranea are fractionated into two equal peaks (16 and 25 s) in a sucrose gradient.
2. After anucleation or after cap formation, the 25 s RNA disappears at a higher rate than the 16 s RNA, which becomes predominant.
3. The pulse-labeled RNA's (17 and 23 s) do not sediment at the same rate as the bulk RNA's (16 and 25 s).
4. Long-term incorporations of H^3-uridine result in an unequal specific radioactivity of the 16 and 25 s RNA's.
5. Chase experiments have shown the existence of a stable 15 s RNA, which is synthesized in the anucleate fragments as well as in the whole plants.

---

[x]Aspirant du Fonds National de la Recherche Scientifique.

17

These results can be interpreted, either by admitting the existence of a non-ribosomal, stable 15 s RNA, or by assuming that several kinds of degradation mechanisms occur in vivo and in vitro, having a preferential action on the 25 s RNA.

Introduction

Anucleate fragments of Acetabularia are capable of regeneration and morphogenesis (Hämmerling, 1953; Brachet et al., 1955). The effects of actinomycin (Brachet et al., 1964; Zetsche, 1964), ribonuclease (Stich and Plaut, 1958) and localized UV-irradiation (Brachet and Olszewska, 1960) suggest that the information needed for these processes might be represented by stable m-RNA molecules, produced by the nucleus and accumulated at the tip of the stalk (Brachet, 1957, 1960). Autoradiographic experiments have shown that labeled precursors of RNA are at first incorporated into the nucleus, and then become distributed along a decreasing apico-basal gradient of concentration (Brachet and Olszewska, 1960; de Vitry, 1963). More direct assays have clearly demonstrated that a gradient of high molecular weight RNA actually exists (Werz, 1960). Ribosomes and polyribosomes are distributed in the same way, as shown by electron microscopy (Werz, 1965, Van Gansen and Boloukhère-Presburg, 1965).

It has been suggested that the chloroplasts, which contain DNA (Baltus and Brachet, 1963; Gibor and Izawa, 1963; Puiseux-Dao et al., 1967) and synthesize RNA (Goffeau and Brachet, 1965; Schweiger et al., 1967; Janowski, 1965; Berger, 1967) might play an important role in morphogenesis, namely by allowing the normal growth of the cap (Brachet et al., 1964; Zetsche, 1964). In appropriate conditions of growth, the anucleate fragments are capable of increasing their net RNA content (Brachet et al., 1964; Schweiger and Bremer, 1961); the chloroplasts are, presumably, the site of this increase, since they contain most of the cellular RNA (Naora et al., 1960). In fact, the chloroplasts and the mitochondria are a complicating factor in the study of RNA metabolism in Acetabularia. Anucleate fragments synthesize chloroplastic (Janowski, 1965, Schweiger et al., 1967), mitochondrial

(Schweiger et al., 1967) and, perhaps, cytoplasmic (post-mitochondrial supernate) (Schweiger et al., 1967) RNA, as well as ribosomes and polyribosomes (Janowski, Bonotto and Bouloukhère, 1969, Baltus et al., 1968). However, some authors have observed a partial or even complete disappearance of rRNA after anucleation (Baltus et al., 1968).

In the present work we have studied, by sucrose gradient sedimentation, the RNA's extracted from Acetabularia mediterranea. We have observed the striking modifications of the sedimentation profiles, after anucleation or after cap formation. We have investigated the characteristics of the pulse-labeled and random-labeled RNA's, as well as the behaviour of the radioactivity during a chase experiment. Finally, we have attempted to present some interpretations of the results.

Material and methods

1. Culture of the algae and incorporation of H^3-uridine.

The algae were cultivated in sterilized sea-water according to Lateur (1963). Incorporation experiments were performed by incubating the plants at room temperature in the presence of H^3-uridine; chase experiments consisted in transferring the plants into a non-radioactive medium, which was changed every day during the first week.

2. Sub-cellular fractions.

Thousand plants or fragments were homogenized in 10 ml (for larger amounts of material, the volume was adapted proportionally) of 0.01 M acetate buffer (pH 5.0) containing 0.54 M glucose, 0.001 M ethylene diamine tetraacetate (EDTA), 1 mg/ml naphtalene disulfonate (NDS) and 100 µg/ml polyvinyl sulfate (PVS). The homogenate was filtered through a piece of bolting silk and centrifuged for 2 min at 70 g (table centrifuge) in order to eliminate the membranes. The chloroplasts were sedimented by a 5 min-centrifugation at 1,200 g and the mitochondria by a 10 min-run at 30,000 g (SS 34-rotor of a Sorvall RC 2 centrifuge). The 30,000 g-supernate is called "cytoplasmic" fraction. The pellets were suspended in 10 ml of the acetate buffer already described. All the manipulations were performed in the cold.

3. Extraction and fractionation of the RNA.

Sodium dodecyl sulfate (SDS) was added to a concentration of 1 % to the total homogenate or to each of the three sub-cellular fractions, which were processed for RNA extraction according to Baltus and Quertier (1966). The final ethanol precipitates were dissolved in a small volume (0.3-0.5 ml) of 0.01 M acetate buffer (pH 5.0) containing 0.001 M EDTA and 20 µg/ml PVS. A same volume of 4.0 M NaCl was added and the mixture was allowed to stand over-night at 4°C. The precipitates were collected by centrifugation and dissolved in 0.3 ml of the acetate buffer containing 0.001 M EDTA and 10 µg/ml PVS. 5-20 % sucrose gradients were centrifuged for 5 hr at 37,500 rpm (or for 3 hr at 45,000 rpm) in the SW 50 rotor of a Spinco L 2 centrifuge. All the operations were performed in the cold. The absorbance at 260 mµ was measured either in diluted fractions, either by collecting the gradients through the flow-cell of a Cary spectrophotometer. The radioactivity of the H^3-uridine-labeled RNA present in the fractions was measured in a liquid scintillation counter (Nuclear, Chicago), using 15 ml of Bray's (1960) solution.

4. Detection of the labeled ribosomes from a total homogenate.

Ten to twenty algae were homogenized in ten times their weight of a 0.01 M Tris-HCl (pH 7.4) solution, containing 0.54 M glucose, 0.01 M KCl, 0.01 M Mg acetate, 0.5 % Na deoxycholate, 0.5% Lubrol and 5 % Triton-X-100. The membrane debris were eliminated by a 5 min- run in a Beckman microfuge (8,500 g). 0.3 ml of the supernate was layered onto a 15-30 % sucrose gradient (buffered at pH 7.4 with 0.01 M Tris-HCl containing 0.01 M Mg acetate) and centrifuged for 2 hr at 45,000 rpm in the SW 50 rotor of a Spinco L2 centrifuge. The TCA- precipitated material, present in the 2 drop-fractions, was collected onto Millipore filters. The radioactivity was measured in the liquid scintillation counter, using 10 ml of the following solution: 5.0 g of 2,5-diphenyloxazole (PPO), 0.5 g of 2,2'-p-phenylene-bis-(4-methyl-5-phenyloxazole (POPOP) in 1 1 of toluene.

Results

1. The behaviour of RNA in nucleate and anucleate cells.

The RNA's extracted from whole, growing Acetabularia mediterranea, are fractionated in two more or less equal peaks in a sucrose gradient (Fig.1a). Analytical ultracentrifugations have shown these RNA's to sediment at 16 and 25 s. When the cap is full-grown, one observes the decrease of the 25 s RNA peak (Fig.1b). The same phenomenon occurs in the case of algae which have been anucleated several days before (Fig.1c). The sedimentation profile of the RNA's extracted from nucleate fragments was not submitted to any change at the time the experiment was performed (25 days after cutting off the stalk) (Fig.1d). Control Escherichia coli radioactive RNA, added to the homogenates of Acetabularia, remained undegraded after the procedure of extraction and purification.

2. The RNA's from the sub-cellular fractions.

The chloroplastic RNA's, which represent 80 % of the cellular RNA content (Naora et al., 1960), display, in a sucrose gradient, the same characteristics as those of the RNA's extracted from a whole homogenate. This has been shown in the case of whole, growing plants (Fig. 2a), of cap-bearing plants (Fig. 2 b) and of anucleate fragments (Fig. 2 c). The RNA's of the mitochondrial fraction (Fig. 2 d) and those of the post-mitochondrial supernate (Fig.2e) have a characteristic sedimentation profile, different from that of the chloroplastic RNA's. We do not know whether cap formation or anucleation has any effect on these sedimentation patterns.

3. Pulse-labeling of the RNA's in nucleate and in anucleate cells.

For convenience, the sedimentation values of the labeled RNA's have been roughly estimated by linear extrapolations. A 30 min-incorporation of H^3-uridine results in the labeling of heterogeneous, slowly sedimenting RNA's and of 17 and 23 s RNA's, as well in whole plants (Fig. 3a) as in anucleate fragments (Fig.3b). The newly synthesized 17 and 23 s RNA's do not sediment at the same rate as the

21

bulk RNA's (16 and 25 s). Though, they appear to be part
of the labeled 30 and 50 s ribosomal particles (Fig. 3 c),
which contain respectively 17 s (Fig. 3d) and 23 s (Fig.
3e) ribosomal RNA.

4. Random labeling of the RNA's in nucleate and in anucleate cells.

Four day-incorporations of H^3-uridine result in the
labeling of the 16 and 25 s bulk RNA's, in whole plants
(Fig. 4a) as well as in anucleate fragments (Fig. 4b).
One should note that, in both the cases, the 25 s RNA displays a higher specific radioactivity than the 16 s RNA.
Moreover, the heterogeneous, slowly sedimenting RNA's,
which were observed after a short-term incorporation of
the labeled precursor, are no longer detectable.

5. Chase labeling of the RNA's in nucleate and in anucleate cells.

Chase experiments have shown that the radioactivity
of the 25 s RNA decreases much more rapidly than that of
the 16 s RNA in the case of whole (Fig. 5a) and of anucleate (Fig. 5b) plants. The 16 s label, which is still present more than two months after the 25 s label has disappeared, is shifted toward a 15 s position in the sucrose
gradient. It is tempting to suggest that this stable, 15
s RNA occurs in a stable 30 s particle, of which the existence has been shown: the sedimentation profile of the 48
hr-labeled particles (Fig. 5c) undergoes striking modifications during a chase experiment. These modifications consist in the disappearance of the 50 s radioactivity; the
30 s label has become predominant after a 20 day-chase
period (Fig. 5d).

6. The chloroplast ribosomes.

Since the 16 and 25 s RNA's of whole, growing plants
do not occur in equimolecular ratio (cf.Fig.2a), it was
interesting to determine the relative amount of the 30 and
50 s chloroplastic ribosomes. They appear to be present in
equimolecular ratio (Fig. 6). We did not succeed in isolating measurable amounts of neither mitochondrial, nor cytoplasmic ribosomes.

Discussion

1. The diversity of RNA species in Acetabularia mediterranea.

       In Acetabularia mediterranea, measurable amounts of
RNA occur in three different classes: on one hand, the mitochondrial and the cytoplasmic (post-mitochondrial supernate) RNA's, displaying the usual sedimentation patterns
of rRNA's (approximately 2:1 surface ratio, corresponding
to equimolecular ratio); on the other hand, the chloroplastic RNA's, which display the same sedimentation profile (approximately 1:1 surface ratio) as the RNA's extracted from whole homogenates. The similarity between the
chloroplastic and the total RNA's is not surprising, since
the chloroplasts contain 80% of the cellular RNA content
(Naora et al., 1960).

2. The relative amount of the 16 and 25 s RNA's.

       In Acetabularia mediterranea, the 16 and 25 s chlo-
roplastic RNA's do not occur in equimolecular ratio. This
fact has been observed in the case of many green plants
(Clark et al., 1964; Spencer and Whitfeld, 1966; Pollard
et al., 1966; Loening and Ingle, 1967; Stutz and Noll,
1967; Oshio and Hase, 1968). Ingle (1968) has shown, in
the case of the radish, this result to be a consequence
of a preferential degradation of the heavier rRNA during
the extraction. Dillard and Schweiger (1969) have suggested that, in the case of Acetabularia, such a degradation
might occur inside the chloroplasts, during the homoge-
neization rather than during the extraction. The latter
hypothesis might explain why control Escherichia coli
RNA, added to Acetabularia homogenates, remains undegraded
after the procedure of extraction. Moreover, Dillard and
Schweiger (this Symposium) succeeded in incresing the 25 to
16 s RNA ratio, by homogenizing the cells at very low temperature. One should note,however,that we obtained equimolecular amounts of 30 and 50 s chloroplastic ribosomal sub-
units. A consequence of Schweiger and Dillard's hypothesis
would be that the 50 s subunits contain partially degraded
25 s RNA. This possibility has not yet been tested.
Another explanation is that the 16 s RNA might have a double nature, only part of it being of true ribosomal origin.

23

3. The behaviour of the RNA's in the absence of the nucleus.

The sedimentation profiles of the RNA's, extracted either from whole homogenates or from chloroplast pellets, undergo striking modifications when the nucleus has been removed. Baltus et al. (1968) have suggested that this phenomenon might be a consequence of the lack of nuclear control. Though, the RNAase content does not increase after anucleation (Schweiger, 1966). Dillard and Schweiger (1969) have observed that the changes of the sedimentation profile of the RNA's occur as soon as one day after anucleation, even in the case of the nucleate fragments; they interpreted this changes as being the result of a trauma-induced degradation of the heavier rRNA. The fact that, in our experiments, the RNA's of the nucleate fragments behave in the same way as those of whole, growing plants, might perhaps be attributed to a repair process during the 25 day-period after surgery.

The sedimentation pattern of the RNA's, extracted from whole homogenates or from the chloroplastic pellet of adult, cap-bearing plants (in which the vegetative nucleus has disappeared), undergoes the same modifications as in the case of anucleate fragments. This observation supports the idea that the nucleus might control the normal level of both the 16 and 25 s RNA's in the chloroplasts. Moreover, Farber et al. (1969) have shown that the ability of the Acetabularia RNA's to stimulate protein synthesis in a cell-free system decreases during cap formation.

The fact that, after anucleation or after cap formation, the 16 and 25 s RNA's disappear at a different rate, might be explained in two different ways, whatever the mechanism may be :
a) the 25 s RNA species is less stable than the 16 s species, which becomes rapidly predominant;
b) both the 16 and 25 s ribosomal RNA's disappear at the same rate, while another, non-ribosomal 16s RNA species becomes predominant because of its relative stability.

4. The pulse-labeled RNA's.

The pulse-labeled RNA's (17 and 23 s) do not sediment at the same rate as the bulk RNA's (16 and 25 s). A first interpretation of this observation might be that the labeled RNA's do not belong to the same sub-cellular fraction as the unlabeled RNA's. However, preliminary experiments (F. Lotstra, unpublished) have suggested that the newly synthesized RNA's do not sediment at the same position as the bulk RNA's, as well in the case of the chloroplastic fraction as in that of the mitochondrial and the post-mitochondrial fractions. Ingle (1968) has observed a similar shift between the radioactivity and the UV-absorbance in the case of the radish; moreover, this author has shown the newly synthesized RNA's not to display the same resistance as the bulk RNA's towards the experimental manipulations. Several interpretations were proposed, namely a change of the spatial configuration of the rRNA's during the ageing of the ribosomes, or to a change of the RNAase content.

5. The random-labeled RNA's.

The 48 hr-labeled RNA's sediment at the same rate as the UV-absorbance. However, the specific radioactivity of the 25 s molecules is higher than that of the 16 s molecules, in the case of whole plants as well as in the anucleate fragments. This fact suggests, that either there is a striking difference between the resistance of the bulk RNA's and the radioactive RNA's toward the manipulations, or a more rapid turn-over of the 25 s RNA, or the existence of an additional species of slowly labeled RNA at the 16 s position.

6. The chase-labeled RNA's.

The chase experiments clearly demonstrate the presence of a stable 15 s RNA species, of which the radioactivity becomes rapidly predominant. On one hand, this 15 s RNA might represent the material which accounts for the unusual sedimentation profile of the Acetabularia RNA's; moreover, it might represent the molecular species which becomes predominant after anucleation or after cap formation; finally its existence might explain the unequal specific radioactivity of the 16 and 25 s RNA's after a 48 hr-incorporation experiment. On the other hand, one might assume the stable 15 s RNA to be the 16 s ribosomal RNA, displaying a lower rate of turnover than the 25 s ribosomal RNA. However, this assumption does not explain the shift of the radioactivity toward the 15 s position during a chase experiment.

The chase-labeled RNA might be part of a stable 30 s particle, of which the existence has been shown. No argument can be presented to decide whether this particle represents the 30 s ribosomal subunit or not.

Conclusions

The RNA's extracted from Acetabularia mediterranea display many puzzling properties:
1) the 16 and 25 s RNA's do not occur in equimolecular amount;
2) the 16 s RNA becomes predominant after anucleation or after cap formation;
3) long-term incorporations (48 hr) of H^3-uridine result in unequal labeling of the 16 and 25 s RNA's;
4) chase experiments show the existence of a stable 15 s RNA, which might be part of a stable 30 s particle.

All these properties might be explained by assuming that the 16 s RNA has a double nature, only part of it being ribosomal. The other part should consist in a special kind of RNA, sedimenting at 15 s and displaying the following properties: stability in the absence of the nucleus, low rate of synthesis and low rate of turnover.

Ruling out the existence of this stable 15 s RNA species needs the accumulation of several assumptions, which do not account for the totality of our observations: a preferential degradation of the 25 s RNA during the manipulations of the homogenates, unequal resistance of the newly synthesized and bulk RNA's toward physical or chemical actions, existence of a trauma-induced degradation of 25 s RNA after surgery, unequal rate of turn-over of the 16 and 25 s RNA's.

Further investigations are needed in order to get information about the nature of the stable 15 s RNA. Perhaps, a thorough study of the base composition of the labeled and unlabeled RNA's sedimenting in the 16 s region might allow us to detect eventual differences between stable and unstable RNA's. Moreover, if some difference exist, one might hope that fractionation of these RNA's is possible by performing polyacrylamide gel electrophoresis or methylated albumin chromatography.

An additional problem in what concerns the properties of the RNA's of Acetabularia arises from the fact that the pulse-labeled RNA's do not sediment at the same rate as the bulk RNA's. One might suggest that the spatial configuration of the r-RNA's undergoes some changes during the ageing of the ribosomes.

Finally, we did not observe appreciable qualitative nor quantitative difference between the behaviour of whole plants and anucleate fragments, as far as the RNA synthesis is concerned. This fact is not surprising, since the chloroplastic DNA content of one Acetabularia is estimated to be 1,000 to 10,000 times higher than the nuclear DNA content (Baltus and Brachet, 1963; Dillard and Schweiger, 1969).

References

Baltus E. and Brachet J. (1963): Biochim. Biophys. Acta, 76, 490.

Baltus E. and Quertier J. (1966) : Biochim. Biophys. Acta, 119, 192.

Baltus E., Edström J.E., Janowski M., Hanocq-Quertier J., Tencer R. and Brachet J. (1968): Proc.N.A.S., 59, 406.

Berger S. (1967) : Protoplasma, 64, 13.

Brachet J. (1957) : Biochemical Cytology, Academic Press, New-York.

Brachet J. (1960): The Biological Role of Nucleic Acids, Elsevier, Amsterdam.

Brachet J. and Olszewska M. (1960) : Nature, 187, 954.

Brachet J., Chantrenne H. and Vanderhaeghe F.(1955) : Biochim. Biophys. Acta, 18, 544.

Brachet J., Denis H. and de Vitry F. (1964) : Develop. Biol., 9, 398.

Bray G.A. (1960): Anal. Biochem., 1, 279.

Clark M.F., Matthews R.E.F. and Ralph R.K. (1964) : Biochim. Biophys. Acta, 91, 289.

de Vitry F. (1963) : Exptl. Cell Res., 31, 376.

Dillard W.L. and Schweiger H.G. (1969) : Protoplasma, 67, 87.

Farber F., Cape M., Decroly M. and Brachet J. (1969): Proc. N.A.S., 61, 843.

Gibor M. and Izawa A. (1963) : Proc.N.A.S., 50, 1164.

Goffeau A. and Brachet J. (1965) : Biochim. Biophys. Acta, 95, 302.

Hammerling J. (1953) : Intern. Rev. Cytol., 2, 475.

Ingle J. (1968) : Plant Physiol., 43, 1448.

Janowski M. (1965) : Biochim. Biophys. Acta, 103, 399.

Janowski M., Bonotto S. and M. Boloukhère (1969) :
Biochim. Biophys. Acta, 174, 525.
Lateur L. (1963) : Revue algolog., 1, 26.
Loening U.E. and Ingle J. (1967): Nature, 215, 363.
Naora H., Naora H. and Brachet J. (1960) : J.Gen. Physiol.,
43, 1083.
Oshio Y. and Hase E. (1968) : Plant & Cell Physiol., 9,
69.
Pollard C.J., Stemler A. and Blaydes D.F. (1966) : Plant
Physiol., 41, 1323.
Puiseux-Dao S., Gibello D. and Hoursiangou-Neubrun D.
(1967) : C.R. Acad. Sc. Paris, 265, 406.
Schweiger H.G., W.L. Dillard, A. Gibor and Berger S.
(1967) : Protoplasma, 64, 1.
Schweiger H.G. and Bremer H.J. (1961): Biochim. Biophys.
Acta, 51, 50.
Spencer D. and Whitfeld P.R. (1966) : Arch. Biochem. Bio-
phys., 117, 337.
Stich H. and Plaut W. (1958) : J.Biophys. Biochem. Cytol.,
4, 119.
Stutz E. and Noll A. (1967) : Proc. N.A.S., 57, 774.
Van Gansen P. and Boloukhère-Presburg M. (1965) : J.
Microsc., 4, 363.
Werz G. (1960) : Planta, 55, 22.
Werz G. (1965) : Planta, 64, 119.
Zetsche K. (1964) : Z.Naturfschg., 19b, 751.

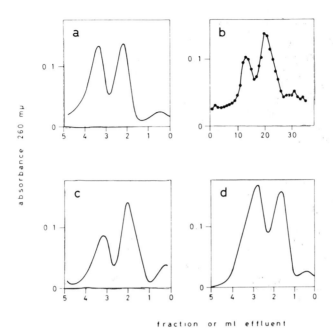

Figure 1. Sucrose gradient sedimentation of the total RNA
extracted from Acetabularia mediterranea.
a) Whole plants.
b) Whole plants bearing a 10 day-old, mature cap.
c) Anucleate fragments, 20 days after surgery.
d) Nucleate fragments, 25 days after surgery.

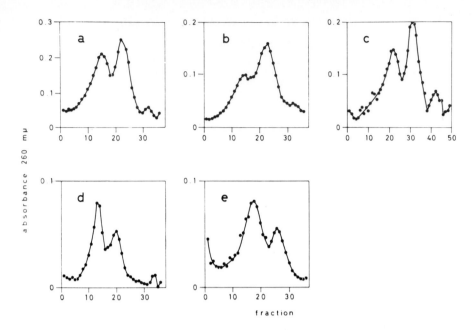

Figure 2. Sucrose gradient sedimentation of the RNA's
        extracted from the sub-cellular fractions of
        Acetabularia mediterranea.
a) Chloroplastic fraction of whole plants.
b) Chloroplastic fraction of whole plants, bearing a 10
   day-old, mature cap.
c) Chloroplastic fraction of anucleate fragments, 5 days
   after surgery.
d) Mitochondrial fraction of whole plants.
e) Cytoplasmic (post-mitochondrial) fraction of whole
   plants.

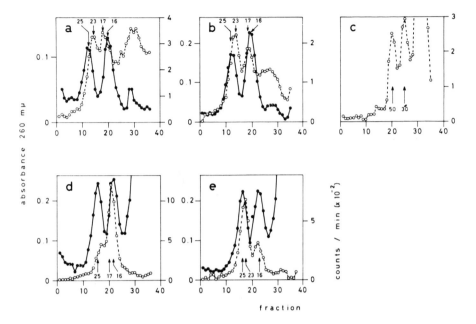

Figure 3. 30 min-incorporation of H³-uridine (20 µc/ml)
into the RNA's and ribosomes of Acetabularia
mediterranea.
a) The RNA's extracted from whole plants.
b) The RNA's extracted from anucleate fragments, 5 days
after surgery.
c) The ribosomes from a total homogenate (whole plants).
d) The RNA extracted from the labeled 30 s ribosomes;
total Acetabularia RNA has been added as a carrier.
e) The RNA extracted from the labeled 50 s ribosomes;
total Acetabularia RNA has been added as a carrier.

●-●-● : absorbance   o-o-o : radioactivity

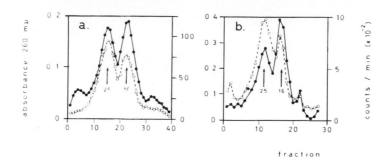

Figure 4. 4 day-incorporation of H^3-uridine (2 μc/ml) into RNA's of <u>Acetabularia mediterranea</u>.
a) The RNA's extracted from whole plants.
b) The RNA's extracted from anucleate fragments, 5 days after surgery.

•-•-• : absorbance   o-o-o : radioactivity

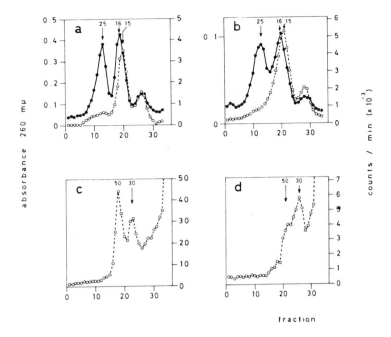

Figure 5. Chase-labeling of the RNA's and ribosomes of
Acetabularia mediterranea.
a) RNA's extracted from whole plants: 6 day-incorporation
of H³-uridine (2 µc/ml), followed by a 34 day-chase.
b) RNA's extracted from anucleate fragments, 25 days
after surgery: 5 day-incorporation of H³-uridine
(2 µc/ml), followed by a 17 day-chase.
c) Ribosomes isolated from whole plants : 2 day-incorporation of H³-uridine (10 µc/ml).
d) Ribosomes isolated from whole plants : 2 day-incorporation of H³-uridine (10 µc/ml) followed by a 20 day-
chase.

●-●-● : absorbance   o-o-o : radioactivity

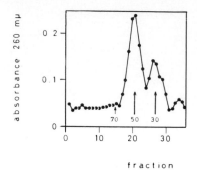

Figure 6. Unlabeled ribosomes isolated from the chloroplastic fraction of whole Acetabularia mediterranea.

THE CYTOPLASMIC DNA'S OF ACETABULARIA MEDITERRANEA : THEIR STRUCTURE AND BIOLOGICAL PROPERTIES

Beverley R. Green and Hugh Burton

Botany Department, University of British Columbia, Vancouver, Canada,

and

Viviane Heilporn and Sylvie Limbosch

Laboratoire de Morphologie Animale, Université Libre de Bruxelles, Brussels, Belgium.

Abstract

Acetabularia mediterranea chloroplast DNA has a buoyant density of 1.704 g/cc, corresponding to 45% GC. It is only partially renaturable, suggesting heterogeneity or very high molecular weight. Mitochondrial DNA is probably the 1.714 g/cc (55% GC) component. Cysts contain chloroplast DNA and another DNA of density 1.697 g/cc (38% GC) in varying proportions. The latter is concluded to be the nuclear DNA.

DNA released by osmotic shock from purified chloroplasts was visualized by the Kleinschmidt technique. Very large amounts of DNA were released from some chloroplasts, whereas others showed smaller amounts apparently attached to the chloroplast lamellae. It is tentatively concluded that Acetabularia chloroplasts probably contain as much DNA as a bacterium, although the information content may not be enough to make them fully autonomous.

Acetabularia has an important place in the history of cytoplasmic DNA. It was one of the first organisms in which it was shown that H3-thymidine was incorporated into the cytoplasm in a DNAase-sensitive form (1). It was also one of the first organisms in which it was shown that isolated chloroplasts contain measurable amounts of DNA (2,3). Because of the ease with which it can be enucleated, it is the only organism in which it can be conclusively shown that the DNA isolated from the chloroplast fraction does not come from contaminating fragments of nuclei (4).

Acetabularia's ability to grow and differentiate without a nucleus has made it one of the most important organisms for the study of nucleocytoplasmic relationships. It is particularly interesting for questions of chloroplast autonomy. D. C. Shephard (5) found that the number of chloroplasts per cell continued to increase after enucleation, although the doubling time increased from 8-9 days to about two weeks. Using autoradiography, he demonstrated that the rate of H3-thymidine incorporation increased at the same rate as the number of chloroplasts in both nucleate and enucleate cells. V. Heilporn-Pohl (6) then estimated the relative amounts of DNA per enucleate alga at various times after enucleation, and found that there was a doubling in the cytoplasmic DNA content over a period of 1-2 weeks. These experiments suggest strongly that the chloroplast DNA replication is independent of the nucleus.

This morning we have heard several exciting papers on the isolation and the synthesis of the various RNA's. It appears that the bulk of RNA synthesis take place in the chloroplast, even in enucleate cells. How much of this RNA synthesis is coded for by the chloroplast DNA is still unknown. It becomes necessary to ask if the chloroplast DNA contains some of the information necessary for the realization of morphogenesis. The fact that an enucleate cell can continue to grow for as long as two months, and can differentiate a cap, suggests that at least some of the genetic information for the growth of the organism may be carried in the DNA of the chloroplast.

In view of the importance of the chloroplast DNA, Drs. Sylvie Limbosch, Viviane Heilporn and myself decided several years ago to make a thorough study of the DNA's of _Acetabularia mediterranea_. We were fortunate in having the excellent collaboration of Dr. Monique Boloukhère, who examined our isolated cell fractions with the electron microscope. Some of this work has already been published (4).

Algae which were 1.5 to 2.5 cm long and had not started to form a cap were treated for several days with a solution of penicillin, neomycin, streptomycin and mycostatin in the concentrations used by Gibor and Izawa (2). They were enucleated and brushed before using. To obtain total cytoplasmic DNA's, about 1000 algae were homogenized gently in several millilitres of 0.4 M mannitol buffered at pH 8.4 and filtered through bolting silk. The filtrate was centrifuged at 12,000 x g for ten minutes and the DNA extracted by the method of Chun, Vaughan, and Rich (7). When the DNA was centrifuged to equilibrium in a CsCl gradient, it was found to contain two bands, at densities of 1.074 and 1.714 g/cc. (Fig. 1). Both of the bands were sensitive to deoxyribonuclease, and both increased in density by 0.016-0.018 g/cc when heat-denatured. (Fig. 3a). The proportions of the two bands varied slightly from one preparation to the next, but there were never more than two peaks and they always had the same density. Similar results were obtained from whole cells, which is not surprising, considering that there are 10^6 to 10^7 chloroplasts for every nucleus, and many of the nuclei would be lost in the homogenization procedure.

For the chloroplast fraction, the bolting-silk filtrate was spun down at 2400 x g for 7 min and washed once with 0.15 M NaCl-0.01 M EDTA, pH 8.5. DNA was isolated as above. The 1.704 g/cc DNA was the main component (Fig.2), with a small amount of the 1.714 g/cc DNA. Electron microscopic examination showed that the fraction consisted of chloroplasts with some mitochondria attached to them. No bacteria were ever observed in this fraction. The same results were obtained in a number of experiments. Similar results were obtained with chloroplasts purified on a sucrose gradient. No matter how the chloroplasts were purified, the 1.704 g/cc peak was always enriched.

Fig.3 (a) shows purified chloroplast DNA denatured by heating to 100°C and quick-cooled. Its density has increased to 1.720 g/cc. Fig. 3 (b) shows partially renatured chloroplast DNA which had been reannealed at 70° for 6 hrs in 2 x SSC at a concentration of 5 µg/ml to a density of 1.710 g/cc. The fact that the renatured DNA did not return to its original density but to an intermediate one suggests either that the DNA is too long to renature properly in 6 hrs, or that is heterogeneous. Wells and

Birnstiel (8) have recently shown that the chloroplast DNA of some higher plants is heterogeneous by its renaturation kinetics.

It has been difficult to get a good preparation of mitochondrial DNA. In this case, it is absolutely essential to work with algae which are very clean, as the bacteria, when present, sediment with the mitochondrial (12,000 x g) fraction. Fig. 4 (b) shows a very small amount of DNA of density 1.714 g/cc from mitochondria purified extensively by a series of differential centrifugations and a DNAase treatment. Other experiments yielded a mixture of the cytoplasmic DNA's, with a relative enrichment of the 1.714 g/cc peaks. However, electron microscope controls have yet to be done. Further evidence in support of this DNA being the mitochondrial DNA comes from the experiments with ethidium bromide treatment which Dr. Limbosch will be reporting later this afternoon.

In order to isolate nuclear DNA, we used either ripe caps or cysts isolated by sterile technique from ripe caps. The caps were washed thoroughly every few days and treated with antibiotics. They were then cut up and the DNA extracted. DNA from caps which had just ripened is shown in Fig. 5. There are two peaks, one at the density of chloroplast DNA and the other at about 1.695 g/cc. When cysts were taken from caps which had been stored in the dark at 10°, then brought into the light for 3 days, the latter peak was much bigger. (Fig. 6). Since at least a month in the dark at lowered temperatures is required for cyst maturation (18), presumably to give the secondary nuclei a chance to divide prior to gamete formation, this suggests that the 1.697 g/cc peak is the nuclear DNA. In fact, when cysts were taken from caps which had undergone dark storage and had then been in the light for 8 days, the DNA was almost exclusively of density 1.697 g/cc. It therefore appears likely that the DNA of lowest density is the nuclear DNA. Our results are summarized in Table 1. The value for gametes was determined by silk-thread electrophoresis (9).

While we were working on this problem, an article by Aharon Gibor appeared in the publication of the Aberystwyth Symposium (10). He had also isolated the chloroplast DNA of <u>Acetabularia</u>, but found a density of 1.695 g/cc. I have discussed the matter with Dr. Gibor, and we are at a loss to explain the divergence in our results. He did not do electron microscopic controls, but he is convinced that the algae used in his experiments were completely bacteria-free. To compound the problem, Dr. Sigrid Berger, working in Dr. Schweiger's laboratory, has found yet a third value for the density of chloroplast DNA. The only explanation I can suggest is that Acetabularia has become so altered by its many years of domestication that strains with different DNA compositions have inadvertantly been selected out.

In support of our results with the Brussels strain of Acetabularia, I should like to point out that we have prepared purified chloroplasts by differential centrifugation at least ten times, and in every case there was only one big peak, and always at a density of 1.704 g/cc. There was usually a small blip at 1.714 g/cc. Several of these preparations were examined by electron microscopy, and in no case were any bacterial profiles found, although there were always mitochondria absorbed to the chloroplasts. It would be rather astonishing if the 1.704 g/cc DNA were due to infecting bacteria, as Dr. Schweiger has suggested, since several species of bacteria are commonly found in the cultures and it would be most unlikely that only one would give up its DNA every time. The yield of DNA from these preparations was about 10 µg per 1000 Acetabularia cells. Assuming a value of 10^{-14} to 10^{-15} g DNA per bacterial cell (Table 2), a yield of 10 µg would require the presence of 10^9 to 10^{10} bacteria, which would form a large grey pellet when first spun down, rather than a small green one. In addition, Dr. Dillard has reported that it makes no difference to his RNA labelling experiments if the algae are not axenic. Since bacterial RNA is more rapidly labelled than chloroplast RNA, it would be surprising if the bacterial DNA made more of a contribution (cold) to the chloroplast DNA than did the hot bacterial RNA to the chloroplast RNA.[x]

---

[x]Footnote. Considerable discussion about the amount of DNA per chloroplast compared to bacteria followed the presentation of this paper. Since it is also relevant to the question of the size of the chloroplast genome, some additional values from the literature have been incorporated into Table 2, and some additional comments made in the text.

I should now like to discuss some of the work I have been doing in Vancouver in collaboration with Mr. Hugh Burton.

The amount of DNA an organelle contains is an indication of how much autonomy it may have. Mycoplasma hominis has the lowest reported DNA content for a bacterium (14). If its 500×10^6 daltons are considered to be the absolute minimum for a free-living organism, then any chloroplast that has at least that much can be considered to have a fair degree of autonomy. The problem of chloroplast genome size is particularly interesting with respect to Acetabularia, which is so strikingly independent of its nucleus. The first published value for its chloroplast DNA content was 10^{-16} or 60×10^6 daltons (2). Dr. Berger has calculated (15) that this would only be enough to code for the ribosomal and transfer RNA's plus about 100 proteins of molecular weight 35-40,000. This is far too few to account for all the enzymes of photosynthesis and protein synthesis, not to mention the actual replication of the chloroplast, which is definitely independent of the nucleus (5).

More recent estimates on Acetabularia and several other chloroplasts put the DNA content within the range of bacterial DNA contents. Some of these are given in Table 2. However, Wells and Birnsteil (8) have shown by renaturation kinetics that lettuce chloroplast DNA consists of two components of 3×10^6 and 120×10^6 daltons. If lettuce is comparable to other higher plants, there are probably a number of these sequences per chloroplast, making the total DNA content much higher, but the actual genome size much more comparable to a viral than a bacterial genome in terms of unique sequences. None of the other chloroplast DNA's has been subjected to this sort of analysis.

As a first step toward the solution of this problem, we have been studying the DNA released from isolated chloroplasts by osmotic shock, using the technique of Kleinschmidt and Zahn (16). Plate 1 is a typical section through a pellet of purified chloroplasts. Approximately one profile in 200 was a mitochondrial profile. No bacteria were seen. The isolated chloroplasts were mixed with cytochrome c in 2M ammonium acetate and layered gently over distilled water. The cytochrome c formed a monolayer at

the air—water interphase, and the chloroplasts were lysed
by the combination of osmotic shock and surface tension.
Some of the released DNA and the chloroplast fragments
were trapped in the monolayer, which was picked up on
Formvar—coated grids. The grids were air—dried and sha-
dowed with a 4:1 mixture of platinum and palladium, first
lightly from all directions, then again from one direction or from two directions at right angles. Shadowing
angle was 7–9°.

Plate 2 shows part of a ruptured chloroplast with
DNA strands apparently attached to the lamellae. DNA–membrane attachments were frequently observed. Some of the
strands in this picture are running parallel, and at one
point seem to be held together by a "blob". This was also
frequently observed. The amount of DNA in this photograph
was measured and found to be 42.7 μ in length, which corresponds to 82×10^6 daltons (26).

The DNA was not always attached to membranes. Plate
3 (a) and (b) are two halves of a composite photo of a
large mass of DNA found close to chloroplast fragments.
No free ends were distinguishable. If you look closely,
you will see that all the "ends" are strands looped back
on themselves. In other words, what we have here is an
enormous amount of supercoiled DNA. I am going to refer
to these masses as "displays" as there is no way to
show whether one or several molecules of DNA are involved.
A free end could easily be hidden in the mass of fibrils.
Displays of this sort were found in every chloroplast
preparation examined.

Plate 4 is an enlargement of part of the display in
Plate 3. The supercoiling is very clearly shown. The diameter of the fibrils at the top of the picture are 70–90A,
which is within the range expected for ordinary duplex, i.
e. double-stranded DNA (27). The tightly supercoiled regions have diameters of about 140 A. In a few spots, fibrils with a diameter of 35–40 A were found, suggesting
the presence of single-stranded regions. However, in each
case there was other material (e.g. stroma) disturbing
the protein monolayer and probably contributing to a
shadowing artifact.

Plate 5 is part of another large display. The un-
coiled region is continuous with the coiled region. Within
the borders of this photo, the linear part of the molecule
measures 17.5 μ and the supercoiled part 57 μ, using a

correction factor of 2.3 for the latter to compensate for loss of length on twisting. This makes a total of 75 μ or 150 x 10^6 daltons for a small part which is only about one-tenth of a display.

In Plate 6, another region of the same display, there is a ring formed by supercoiling. The same result can be obtained by twisting a piece of string until it starts to form loops, then letting it go slowly. Note that the DNA disappears into a mass of stroma but appears to re-emerge.

It should be noted that the fact that the DNA is supercoiled does not mean it is circular. A very long molecule (or piece of string) can easily retain one or several twists in the same or opposite direction while being free to rotate, simply because of its very great length. This is the basis of one of the most recent models of chromosome replication (28).

About 20% of the chloroplast fragments had DNA either attached to them or in the vicinity. Presumably the rest had been ejected into the hypophase or trapped under fragments of lamellae. The nature of the attachment to the membranes is unknown. It could be a reflection of in vivo attachment, or it could be fortuitous. Similar attachments have been found by other workers in Acetabularia, (29) higher plants, (30) and the brown alga Sphacelaria (31). We have found them in chloroplasts from another siphoneous green alga, Halicystis parvula. This alga is multinucleate, so the nuclei cannot be separated except by differential centrifugations and a DNAase treatment. Plate 7 shows the DNA of a lysed chloroplast, apparently attached to the membrane. The total length of the DNA is 54.2 μ. We did not see any displays, probably because of the presence of a small amount of residual DNAase.

In none of our experiments have we seen any of the "mesh" DNA of Fernandez-Moran and Woodcock (30). Perhaps the DNA of higher plant chloroplasts is different, but I suspect that their "mesh" DNA is a shadowing artifact due to the presence of stroma. Neither have we seen any of the "looped" single-stranded DNA seen by Werz and Kellner (29).

Unfortunately, supercoiled molecules are not the best material on which to measure length. We are now looking for methods of disrupting chloroplasts and "relaxing" the DNA without breaking it. Preliminary measurements of five molecules from chloroplasts lysed by gentle shaking

with sarkosyl and phenol are given in Table 3, along with
the measurements of parts of displays. Many of the molecules in this preparation were broken into short pieces, and
there were quite a few which appeared to be denatured. The
long molecules measured have probably also been degraded,
as they are the same size as small regions of the "displays".
Taken together, these results suggest that the size of the
chloroplast DNA genome is much greater than the 60×10^6
daltons originally estimated.

Summary

The chloroplast, mitochondrial, and nuclear DNA of
Acetabularia mediterranea have been isolated and identified on the basis of their buoyant densities of 1.704,
1.714, and 1.697 g/cc respectively. Very large amounts of
DNA are released from chloroplasts lysed by osmotic shock.
Preliminary estimates indicate there must be at least
150×10^6 daltons of DNA per chloroplast, and probably
much more. This brings the DNA content up to a quantity
which would be sufficient for a free-living organism.
This question is being investigated further. However, it
will also be necessary to determine the size of the unique
sequences, or actual information content, by renaturation
experiments. (32).
It still remains to be shown what functions the
chloroplast DNA has. Is it simply a self-reproducing machi-
ne for photosynthesis, or is it involved in morphogenesis?
It seems to me that little further progress can be made in
understanding morphogenesis until the techniques of genetics are brought to bear on this organism. I fully realize
what difficulties are involved in any genetic work on
Acetabularia, but if every research group represented in
this room were to set itself the task of isolating two
or three mutants, we would soon have enough to start answe-
ring some of the outstanding questions in development.

References

1. J. Brachet, Exp. Cell Res. 6, 78 (1958).
2. A. Gibor and M. Izawa, Proc. U.S. Nat. Acad. Sci. 50, 1164 (1963).
3. E. Baltus and J. Brachet, Biochim. Biophys. Acta 61, 157 (1963).
4. B. R. Green, V. Heilporn, S. Limbosch, M. Boloukhère and J. Brachet, Proc. U.S. Nat. Acad. Sci. 58, 1351 (1967).
5. D. C. Shephard, Exp. Cell Res. 37, 93 (1965).
6. V. Heilporn-Pohl and J. Brachet, Biochim. Biophys. Acta, 119, 429 (1966).
7. E.H.L. Chun, M.L. Vaughan and A. Rich, J. Mol. Biol. 7, 130 (1963).
8. R. Wells and M. Birnstiel, Biochem. J. 112, 777 (1969).
9. E. Baltus, J. Edstrom, M. Janowski, J. Hanocq-Quertier, R. Tencer and J. Brachet, Proc. U.S. Nat. Acad. Sci. 59, 406 (1968).
10. A. Gibor, in "Biochemistry of the Chloroplasts", ed. T.W. Goodwin. Acad. Press, N.Y. 1967. Vol. 2, p. 321.
11. C. Mereschowsky, Biol. Zbl. 25, 593 (1905).
12. M. M. K. Mass, Science 165, 25 (1969).
13. S. Granick and A. Gibor, Prog. Nuc. Acid Res. Mol. Biol. 6, 143 (1967).
14. R. Bode and H. Morowitz, J. Mol. Biol. 23, 191 (1967).
15. S. Berger, Protoplasma 64, 13 (1967).
16. A. K. Kleinschmidt and R.K. Zahn, Z. Naturforschung 14b, 730 (1959).
17. Calculated using the values for number of chloroplasts/ alga given by Shephard (5).
18. L. Lateur, Rev. Algol. 1, 26 (1963).
19. T. Iwamura and S. Kuwashima, Biochim, Biophy. Acta 174, 330 (1969).
20. G. Brawerman and J.M. Eisenstadt, Ibid. 91, 477 (1964).
21. S.D. Kung and J.P. Williams, Biochim. Biophys. Acta 169, 265 (1968).
22. W.D. Cooper and H.L. Loring, J. Biol. Chem. 228, 813 (1957).
23. J. Cairns, J. Mol. Biol. 6, 208 (1963).
24. I.W. Craig, C.K. Leach, N.G. Carr, Arkiv. Mikrobiol. 65, 218 (1969).

25. P.C. Caldwell & C. Hinshelwood, J. Chem. Soc. 1950, p. 1415.
26. M.H.F. Wilkins, Science 140, 941 (1963).
27. A.K. Kleinschmidt, in Methods in Enzymology. Vol. 12B, p. 361 (ed. L. Grossman and K. Moldave).
28. C. Person and D.T. Suzuki, Can. J. Gen. Cytol. 10, 627 (1968).
29. G. Werz and G. Kellner. J. Ult. Res. 24, 109 (1968).
30. C.L.F. Woodcock and H. Fernandez-Moran, J. Mol. Biol. 31, 627 (1968).
31. T. Bisalputra and H. Burton. J. Ult. Res., in press.
32. R.J. Britten and D.E. Kohne, Science 161, 529 (1968).

Acknowledgements

This work was supported by the National Research Council of Canada and the Fonds National de la Recherche Scientifique Belge. We would like to thank Mr. L. Lateur and Mr. J. Verhulst for their excellent technical assistance, and Dr. T. Bisalputra for helpful advice and the use of the Zeiss EM 9A electron microscope.

Table 1.

THE DNA's OF ACETABULARIA MEDITERRANEA

Enucleate Cells	ρ(g/cc)	% GC.
Chloroplasts	1.704	45
Mitochondria	1.714	55
Cysts	1.697	38
	1.704	45
Gametes	–	42

Table 2.

DNA CONTENT OF CHLOROPLASTS[1] AND BACTERIA

	Wt(x10^16g)	Mol. Wt. (daltons x10^6)	Estimated Length (μ)	Ref.
(a) Chloroplasts of :				
Acetabularia mediterranea	1	60	30	2
	3-4	180-240	90-120	13
	1-10	60-600	30-300	13
	10-50	600-3000	300-1500	17
Chlorella ellipsoidea	40	2400	1200	19
Euglena gracilis	110	6600	3300	20
Vicia faba	57	3400	1700	21
Nicotiana tabacum	80	4800	2400	22
(b) Bacteria and Blue-green Algae.				
Escherichia coli	50	3000	1500	23
Aerobacter aerogenes	20	1200	600	25
Mycoplasma hominis	-	500	250	14
Anacystis nidulans	300	1800	9000	24

[1]Assuming chloroplast genome all in one piece (26).

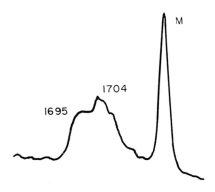

Fig. 5: Cyst DNA from newly-ripened caps.

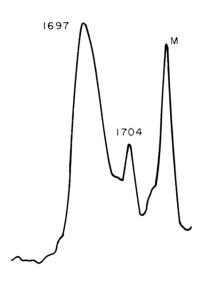

Fig. 6: DNA from caps stored at 10°C then exposed to light for 3 days at 20°C.

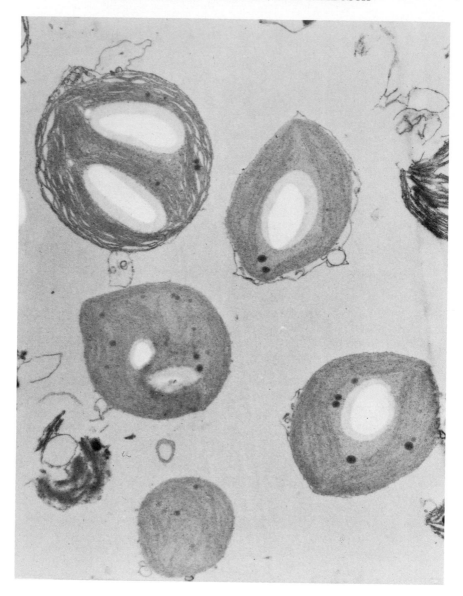

Plate 1. Isolated chloroplasts fixed in
glutaraldehyde, posfixed with
OsO4 and embedded in Maraglas.
(21,600X).

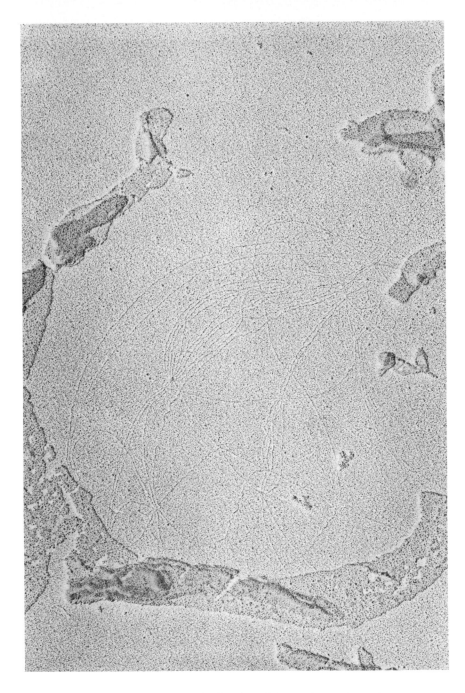

Plate 2.   <u>Acetabularia</u> chloroplast lysed
           by osmotic shock.
           (34,560X).

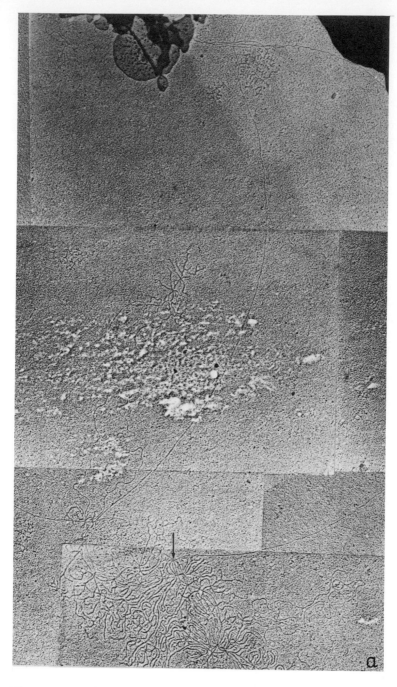

Plate 3.　(a) and (b) Composite of "display" of DNA (22,320X).

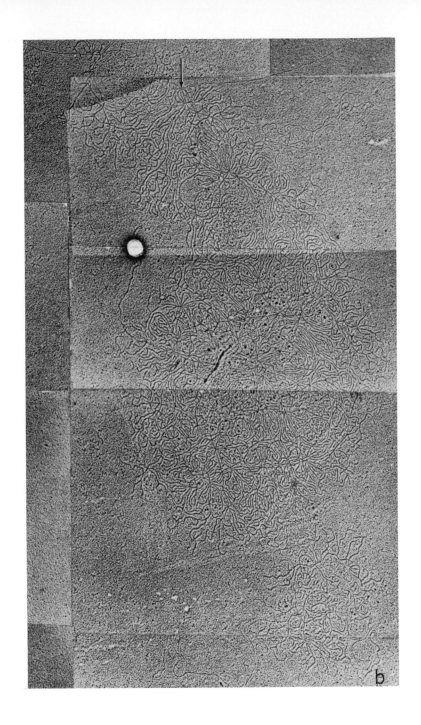

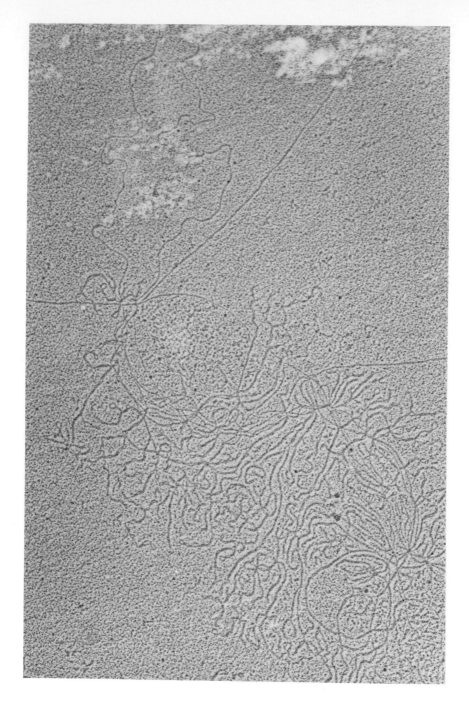

Plate 4.   Enlargement of part of Plate 3. Note
            supercoiling. (40,320X).

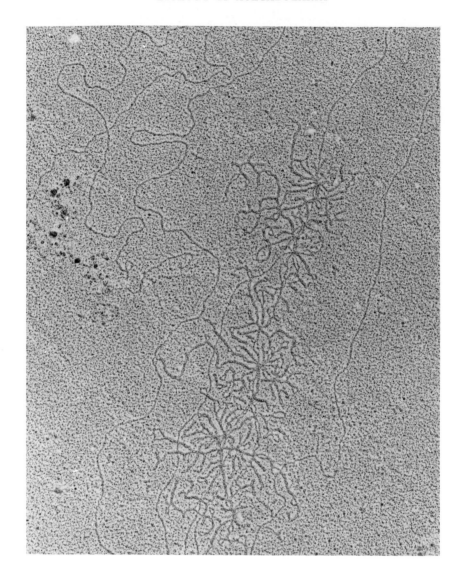

Plate 5.   Part of a large "display". Note
supercoiling. (18,360X).

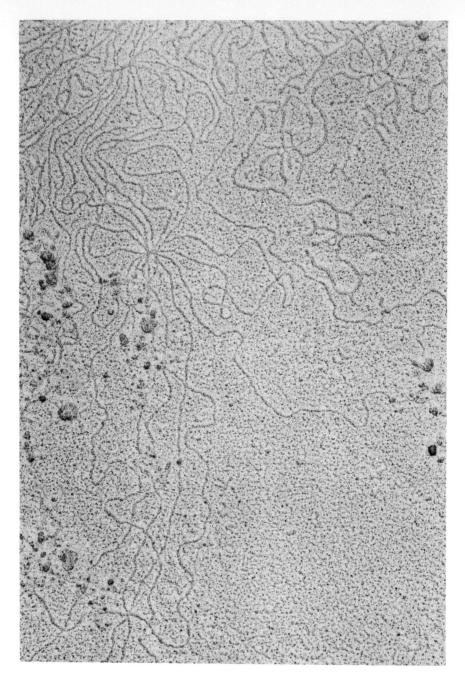

Plate 6.   Part of the same "display" as Plate 5.
Ring is found on middle left side.
(54,000X).

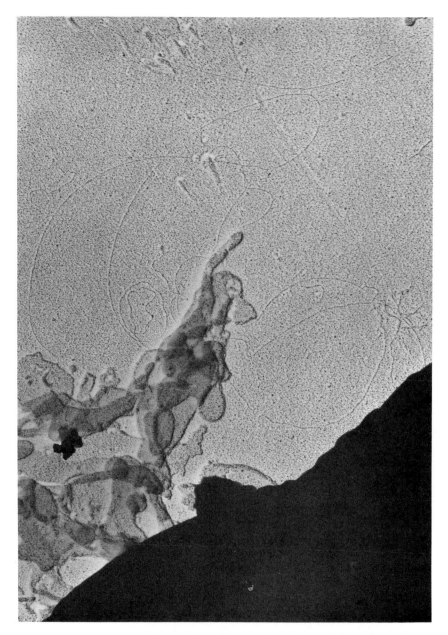

Plate 7.　Halicystis chloroplast lysed by osmotic shock. (32,922X).

EFFECTS OF HYDROXYUREA AND ETHIDIUM BROMIDE ON ACETABULARIA MEDITERRANEA

Viviane Heilporn[x] and Sylvie Limbosch[x]

Laboratoire de Morphologie Animale
Université Libre de Bruxelles,
Brussels, Belgium.

Abstract

The effects of hydroxyurea, an inhibitor of DNA synthesis, and ethidium bromide, an intercalating dye in nucleic acids, on the morphogenesis, the synthesis of nucleic acids and the density of the cytoplasmic DNAs have been studied in nucleate and anucleate fragments of Acetabularia mediterranea.
Hydroxyurea. It was found that
1) the morphostatic effect of hydroxyurea is most marked at the beginning of cap formation,
2) in the presence of hydroxyurea, the synthesis of nucleic acids in the cytoplasm is inhibited in the whole algae as well as in anucleate fragments,
3) in our hands, no modification ever occurred of the density of the cytoplasmic DNAs, as a result of treatment with hydroxyurea.
Ethidium bromide. The results have shown that, in the presence of ethidium bromide
1) the morphogenesis of the algae is blocked,
2) the cytoplasmic DNA synthesis is completely inhibited after 8 and 15 days treatment,
3) the mitochondrial DNA peak, obtained in cesium chloride gradient (density: 1.714 g/cc), disappears almost completely ; chloroplast DNA (density : 1.704 g/cc) is, on the

---

x Chargées de Recherches au Fonds National de la Recherche Scientifique.

other hand, found in both treated and control plants,
4) the cytochrome oxydase activity is reduced. All these
inhibitory effects are partially reversible by transfer
of the treated algae to normal sea water.

Introduction

In order to complete the study of cytoplasmic DNAs
of Acetabularia, we have studied the effects of two substances which are well known for their inhibiting action
on DNA synthesis : hydroxyurea, a strong inhibitor of the
DNA synthesis in all kinds of biological materials (1-5),
and ethidium bromide, a phenantridine drug which forms soluble metachromatic complexes with nucleic acids (6).

1. The effects of hydroxyurea

The mechanism of action of hydroxyurea is not yet
fully understood. Many hypotheses have been advanced on
this subject. For instance, it has been suggested that
hydroxyurea may inhibit the reduction of ribonucleotides
(1-5); on the other hand, it might produce changes in the
DNA molecule itself (7). According to Vogler, Bain and
Huguley (8), hydroxyurea may prevent the synthesis of pyrimidines.
It therefore seems interesting to study the effects
of hydroxyurea on the cytoplasmic DNAs of Acetabularia.
DNA synthesis certainly occurs in anucleate fragments (9),
and is probably related to the multiplication of chloroplasts and mitochondria. We have therefore studied the effects of hydroxyurea upon the synthesis, the metabolism
and the density of cytoplasmic DNAs.

Methods

The effects of hydroxyurea upon the cytoplasmic
DNAs of Acetabularia have been studied in three ways:
a) the DNA content of control algae as compared with spe-
cimens treated with hydroxyurea (0.1 and 0.3 mg/ml) has
been estimated by the fluorometric method of Kissane and

Robbins (10), as modified by Baltus and Brachet (11).
b) the incorporation of ^{3}H-uridine (specific radioactivity:
5000 mC/mM) into DNA and RNA was measured by scintillation
counting, as previously described (12).
c) the effects of hydroxyurea upon the density of cytoplasmic DNAs has been followed by ultracentrifugation in cesium chloride of DNA extracted, from treated and control
algae, by a slight modification of Marmur's method (13).
Centrifugations were carried out at 44,000 rpm, for 24
hours, in an AN-D rotor (Spinco, model E).

Results

The most striking morphostatic effect of hydroxyurea at concentrations of 0.1 and 0.3 mg/ml appears at the
time when the reproductive cap of the algae is about to be
formed, as has already been shown by the work of Brachet
(14). This effect is largely reversible : it is enough to
return the algae to normal sea water and 50 % of pretreated plants regain their ability to form a cap.
The effects of hydroxyurea on the synthesis of cytoplasmic DNAs in both nucleate and anucleate fragments
have been studied. The results obtained after 7 and 15
days of treatment are given in figure 1. It can be seen
that hydroxyurea very markedly reduces the synthesis of
cytoplasmic DNAs. When the algae were returned to normal
sea water, DNA synthesis resumes though at a lower rate
than before.
In order to check a hypothesis of Yarbro (15), suggesting that hydroxyurea probably inhibits the reduction
of ribonucleotides, we have added NADPH (0.2 mg/ml) to the
hydroxyurea solutions used to treat the algae. Fluorometric assays show (see figure II) that this addition results in a relatively higher rate of the DNA synthesis,
although, paradoxically, growth and morphogenesis are not
similarly improved.
The incorporation of ^{3}H-uridine into the DNA and
RNA of the treated and control algae has been further
studied in the presence and absence of hydroxyurea : the
result was an inhibition of the incorporation of uridine,
DNA synthesis being more affected than RNA synthesis
(see figure III).

Finally we attempted to verify the observations made by Rosenkranz (16) and Bendich and al. (17) who were able to demonstrate a direct effect of hydroxyurea on the structure of bacterial DNA. We were unable to obtain similar results with Acetabularia : treatment with hydroxyurea, at various concentrations (0.1 and 0.3 mg/ml), and for varying times (4 and 6 days), did not alter the density in cesium chloride gradients of the extracted DNA. The figure IV illustrates the results obtained under our experimental conditions (12) : the two peaks of chloroplastic (1.704 g/cc) and mitochondrial (1.714 g/cc) DNA are found both in control and treated plants.

Discussion

These findings clearly demonstrate that hydroxyurea inhibits the synthesis of DNA in both nucleate and anucleate fragments. In the latter case, the inhibitor is probably acting upon the cytoplasmic synthesis which, in the absence of the nucleus, ensures the multiplication of the chloroplasts (and of the mitochondria), the growth of the algae and the formation of the cap.

Hydroxyurea did not affect the structure of the cytoplasmic DNAs under the experimental conditions we have used. These results do not necessarily contradict those of Rosenkranz (16), since this author had to use lethal doses of hydroxyurea in order to obtain structural modifications of bacterial DNA.

The data presented here do not furnish an explanation of the mechanism of action of hydroxyurea, nor do they permit a choice between the several hypotheses already proposed. The fact that the incorporation of thymidine is only slightly reduced by hydroxyurea, even after 4 days treatment, whereas the level of synthesis of DNA is increased when NADPH is added at the same time as hydroxyurea, supports the idea that the reduction of ribonucleotides to deoxyribonucleotides is inhibited by this reagent (15). However, this does not explain the inhibition, by hydroxyurea, of uridine incorporation into RNA.

2. The effects of ethidium bromide

The phenantridine compound, ethidium bromide, has been used extensively as trypanocidal agent ; its pharmacological effectiveness must be partially based on its intercalation between the base pairs of DNA molecules. This intercalation alters the structure of the nucleic acids and has facilitated the separation of molecules of mitochondrial DNA from those of nuclear origin (18).

The work of Steinert et al. (19) has shown that ethidium bromide specifically inhibits the replication of kinetoplastic DNA of trypanosomes, that is to say, that of mitochondrial DNA.

Recently, it has been shown, that ethidium bromide induces mutants of yeast (which are called "ρ-petites") by a change in the buoyant density of their mitochondrial DNA (20).

Therefore it seemed interesting to look for a similar specific action of ethidium bromide on mitochondrial DNA in Acetabularia.

Methods

We have studied the effects of ethidium bromide on the synthesis of cytoplasmic DNAs both in nucleate and anucleate fragments, using the sensitive fluorometric method (10-11). The density in cesium chloride gradient of cytoplasmic DNAs extracted from control and treated algae has also been compared (13). Finally, we measured the activity of cytochrome oxydase in control and treated cells using the method of Cooperstein et al. (21). These estimations have been made on mitochondrial enriched fractions (13) extracted from about 150 algae.

Results

The morphological observations made by Brachet (22) have been confirmed. In the presence of ethidium bromide, at concentrations of 20 and 30 µg/ml, the nucleate and anucleate fragments lose their hair whorls after 3 days treatment ; no regeneration is observed in the treated

algae, nor does one observe even the initiation of a reproductive cap. These effects are reversible when the algae are returned to sea water. Ethidium bromide however
becomes lethal if a continuous treatment is pursued for
more than 20 days.

DNA synthesis is inhibited in the nucleate and anucleate fragments after treatment with ethidium bromide.
The figure V shows that the DNA content remains constant,
whereas it doubles in the control after 8 days of culture.
A simple transfer for 8 days, of the treated algae to normal sea water is followed by a renewal of DNA synthesis.

The densities in cesium chloride gradients of cytoplasmic DNAs extracted from control and treated algae have
been compared. It can be seen on figure VI (A and B) that,
after 5 days treatment with ethidium bromide (25 µg/ml),
the mitochondrial peak, with a density of 1.714 g/cc,
disappears almost completely. On the other hand, the chloroplastic DNA, density of which is 1.704, is found both in
treated and control algae. Again this effect is reversible
by a simple transfer of treated algae into normal sea
water (see figure VI, C).

Since ethidium bromide seems to affect preferential-
ly the mitochondrial DNA of the algae, we measured the activity of cytochrome oxydase in control and treated algae.
The results, illustrated in the figure VII, show that ethidium bromide inhibits the activity of cytochrome oxydase
and that the inhibitory effect is partially reversible
when the algae are put back into normal sea water.

Discussion

To conclude, the fluorometric assays of DNA demonstrate that replication of cytoplasmic DNA is almost completely inhibited in the treated algae. This inhibition
probably results from the ethidium bromide intercalation
between the two strands of chloroplastic and mitochondrial
DNAs.

In order to explain the disappearence, after 4
days treatment with ethidium bromide, of the peak 1.714,
which is presumed to be mitochondrial DNA, it is tempting
to suggest that the mitochondria of Acetabularia are fairly short-lived, and that their DNA is quickly replicated.

Since ethidium bromide prevents any replication of DNA, the genetic material of mitochondria would finally be lost. The reappearance of mitochondrial DNA, in algae treated for 4 days with ethidium bromide, then returned for 15 days to normal sea water, would be due to the renewed synthesis of mitochondrial DNA using the few remaining intact copies. The inhibition of the activity of cytochrome oxydase, a mitochondrial enzyme, in the presence of ethidium bromide, is in agreement with this hypothesis.

Our results seem to show a certain parallelism with those of Steinert et al. (19) who studied the disappearence of the kinetoplast in trypanosomes treated with ethidium bromide ; this fact would result from the preferential inhibition of the replication of kinetoplast DNA and from the dilution of this DNA in the course of the cell division which follows the beginning of the treatment. Whether a similar explanation holds true for the mitochondrial population in Acetabularia, could be established by an ultrastructural analysis of the treated algae.

Acknowledgements

We wish to thank Dr. P. Malpoix for the translation of the manuscript and L. Lateur and J. Verhulst for expert technical assistance. We are deeply gratified to Mrs E. De Saedeleer for the photographs.

References

1. J.W. Yabro, B.J. Kennedy and C.P. Barnum, Proc.Natl. Acad. Sci. 53, 1033, (1965).
2. R. Adams, R. Abrams and I.J. Lieberman, J. Biol. Chem. 241, 903, (1966).
3. C. Young and S. Hodas, Science 146, 1172, (1964).
4. M. Turner, R. Abrams and I. Lieberman, J. Biol. Chem. 241, 5777, (1966).
5. L.S. Cohen and G.P. Studzinski, J. Cellular Comp. Physiol. 69, 331, (1967).
6. M.J. Waring, Biochim. Biophys. Acta 114, 234, (1966).
7. H.S. Rosenkranz and H.S. Carr, J. Bacteriol. 92, 178 (1966).

8. W.R. Vogler, J.A. Bain and C.M. Huguley, Proc.Am. Assoc. Cancer Res. 6, 592, (1965).
9. V. Heilporn and J.Brachet, Biochim. Biophys. Acta 119, 429, (1966).
10. J. Kissane and E. Robbins, J. Biol. Chem. 233, 184, (1958)
11. E. Baltus and J. Brachet, Biochim. Biophys. Acta 76, 490, (1963).
12. V. Heilporn-Pohl and S. Limbosch-Rolin, Biochim. Biophys. Acta 174, 220, (1969).
13. B. Green, V. Heilporn, S. Limbosch, M. Boloukhère and J. Brachet, Proc. Natl. Acad. Sci. 58, 1351, (1967).
14. J. Brachet, Nature 214, 1132, (1967).
15. J.W. Yarbro, J. Clin. Invest. 45, 1090, (1966).
16. H.S. Rosenkranz, Biochim. Biophys. Acta 129, 618, (1966).
17. A. Bendich, E. Borenfreund, G.C. Korngold, M. Krim and M.E. Balis, Acidi Nucleici e loro Funzione Biologica, Convegno Antonio Baselli, Milano, (1963), Tipografia Successori Fusi, Pavia, 214, (1964).
18. R. Radloff, W. Bauer and J. Vinograd, Proc. Natl. Acad. Sci. 57, 1514, (1967).
19. M. Steinert, S. Van Assel and G. Steinert, Exp. Cell Res. 56, 69, (1969).
20. P. Slonimski, G. Perrodin and J. Croft, Biochem. and Biophys. Res. Comm. 30, 232 (1968).
21. S.J. Cooperstein and A. Lazarow, J. Biol. Chem. 189, 665, (1951).
22. J. Brachet, Nature 220, 488, (1968).

Figure 1.

Effects of hydroxyurea (HU) on the DNA content per whole and anucleate alga.

Exp.	Days of treatment	Control	Whole algae HU 0.1mg/ml	HU 0.3mg/ml	Anucleate algae Control	HU 0.1 mg/ml
I	0	15	–	–	12	–
	8	24 (+61%)	14 (-6%)	17 (+16%)	20 (+71%)	12 (+4%)
II	0	24	–	–	21	–
	8	30 (+22%)	23 (-4%)	24 (0%)	31 (+45%)	22 (+2%)

The results are expressed as mµg of DNA per alga . The percentage stimulation or inhibition as compared with controls at 0 time is also indicated.

Figure II.

Effects of hydroxyurea (HU) and hydroxyurea + NADPH on whole algae DNA content.

Days of treatment	Control	HU 0.3 mg/ml	HU (0.3 mg/ml) + NADPH (0.2 mg/ml)
0	84	–	–
7	115 (+36%)	86 (+2%)	103 (+21%)

The results are expressed as mµg of DNA per alga. The percentage stimulation or inhibition as compared with controls at 0 time is also indicated.

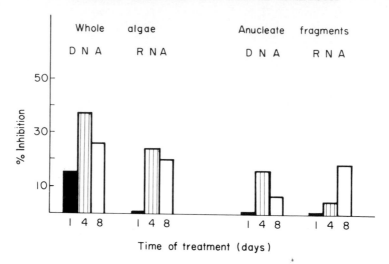

Figure III.

Inhibition of the incorporation of ^{3}H uridine into the DNA and into the RNA of algae treated with hydroxyurea (0,1 mg/ml).

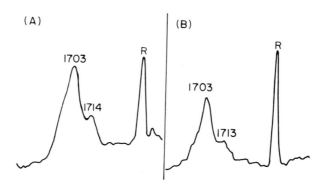

Figure IV.

CsCl density gradient centrifugation of DNA from anucleate fragments of Acetabularia.
A : Control DNA
B : DNA of algae treated by hydroxyurea (0.1 mg/ml) for 4 days (R = LP7 phage DNA reference, density : 1.741 g/cc).

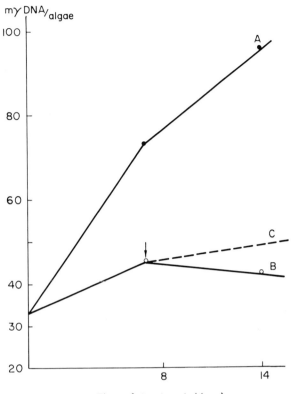

Figure V.

Effects of ethidium bromide on the synthesis of DNA in
anucleate fragments of <u>Acetabularia</u>.
A : Control algae.
B : Algae treated with ethidium bromide (25 µg/ml)
C : Algae treated for 7 days and transfered to sea water
for 7 days.

71

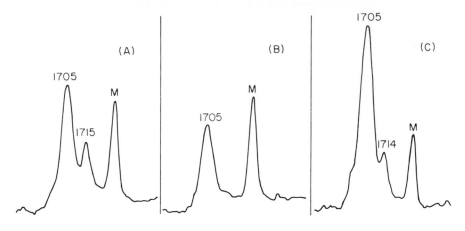

Figure VI.

CsCl density gradient centrifugations of cytoplasmic
DNAs of:
A : Control algae.
B : Ethidium bromide treated algae (25 μg/ml) for 4 days.
C : Algae treated for 4 days and transfered to sea water
    for 15 days.
    (M : Micrococcus lysodeikticus DNA reference, density:
    1.731 g/cc).

Figure VII.

Percentage inhibitium of cytochrome oxydase activity in
algae treated with ethidium bromide (25 μg/ml).

	Experiments			
	I	II	III	IV
				normal sea water
days of treatment	5	8	5	4 ⟶ 6
% inhibition	50	59	52	38 11

THE FINE STRUCTURE OF THE GAMETES AND ZYGOTES OF ACETABULARIA[x]

J.C.W. Crawley

Medical Research Council,
Clinical Research Centre,
Radioisotopes Division,
Guy's Hospital Medical School,
London, England

Abstract

The two flagella of the gamete of Acetabularia enter the cell through a raised portion of the cell membrane and have roots near the cell surface. A large peripheral chloroplast contains the eyespot, but no connection was seen between this organelle and the roots of the flagella. The two eyespots of the zygote did not assume a recognisable relationship at a stage that was early enough to account for the negative phototaxis. The two nuclei of the zygote remained almost in contact whilst bridges formed between the nuclear membranes.

Introduction

Acetabularia is one of the few unicellular organisms to be studied before microscopes were generally available. Parkinson (1) discussed the possible therapeutic value of a plant he called "Umbilicus marinus", which from his line drawing (fig.1) is clearly Acetabularia mediterranea. In recent years the importance of this organism as an experimental material for cell biology (2) has made its fine structure a subject of great interest. Initial difficulties

---

[x] The work described here was carried out in the Department of Cell Biology of the John Innes Institute.

with fixation (3,4) have now been overcome, and there have been electron microscope studies of a number of stages of the developing cell. The gametes and zygotes of <u>Acetabularia</u> have some interesting features. There is a sudden change from positive to negative phototaxis when gametes fuse, and the nuclei fuse to form a nucleus which does not divide until it is the giant nucleus of a mature cell. A sharp contrast to the situation in most organisms where a division occurs soon after the nuclei from the gametes fuse.

In some algae the chloroplasts from one gamete degenerate soon after fusion (5). De Bary and Strassburger (6) showed the gametes of <u>Acetabularia</u> with large pale chloroplasts and the zygotes with small denser chloroplasts, so any changes in chloroplast structure soon after fusion are not of great interest.

The work described here is a survey of the fine structure of gametes and zygotes intended as a foundation for more detailed studies.

Material and Methods

Cysts of <u>Acetabularia crenulata</u> and <u>Acetabularia mediterranea</u> were subjected to osmotic shock and placed in a shallow dish of Erdschreiber medium under oblique illumination. When gametes were released they were transferred from the light side of the dish to the top layer of a centrifuge tube of Erdschreiber solution illuminated from above. The negatively phototaxic zygotes sank to the bottom of the tube and were fixed at various times up to 16 hours by replacing the Erdschreiber medium with 6% gluteraldehyde buffered with cacodylate buffer. This method gave only an approximate time after fusion because some gametes may have fused some time after their transfer. Gametes were fixed by transferring them in a pipette with a small drop of medium to a centrifuge tube of fixative and gently centrifuging to produce a pellet.

Observations and Discussion

Gametes

The two flagella join the cell obliquely in a raised portion and have roots which continue just inside the

cell membrane (fig. 2). No connection was seen between
the roots of the flagella and the eyespot, an ordered array
of dense globules (fig.3), but a very lucky section would
be required to reveal such a connection. The eyespot was
always found near the surface of the cell (fig. 3) and in
a large chloroplast which covered much of the periphery
(fig. 4). Smaller chloroplasts and mitochondria were also
observed. The internal structure of the chloroplasts was
rather sparse, with small thylacoids, each containing only
a few lamellae. The nucleus has a typical double membrane,
but the spacing between the membranes was not uniform
(fig. 2). This may be due to damage in fixation, but it
occurs in gametes and early zygotes and not in cells a few
millimetres long; it may therefore reflect a feature of
the nucleus at this stage of development. No nucleolus
was observed, but densely stained areas occurred in all
sections of nuclei (figs. 2 and 4).

Zygotes

Very early zygotes were difficult to prepare for
the electron microscope, possibly because the cell membranes must break during fusion. Some sections (fig. 5)
showed early contact between gametes with two cells just
merging. When such sections were found the cell membrane
was missing, but this was probably an artifact of fixation due to the fragile nature of the cells at this stage.
Where the cytoplasm had started to fuse (fig. 6) trans-
verse and longitudinal sections of flagella (or the roots
of flagella) could be seen. At this stage the cytoplasm
appeared very rich in ribosomes, possibly a reflection of
intense metabolic activity.

There was no immediate contact between the two eyespots, so the change from positive to negative phototaxis
remains unexplained. At a later stage, too late to account for the change in phototaxis, the two chloroplasts
with eyespots came close together and at a later stage
the two eyespots appeared to be in one chloroplast.
This may be an illusion due to sectioning degenerating
eyespots, but the implications of fusing chloroplasts are
important. It should be possible to confirm or support
this view by labelling some gametes with radioactive compounds and studying the sections by autoradiography (7).

The two nuclei come close together and remain almost in contact whilst bridges form between the nuclear membranes (8). The statistical method used in that paper to analyse the pictures of nuclei seen in zygotes has since been tested on a system consisting of synchronously dividing yeast (9).

The layer of cytoplasm closely applied to the surface of the nuclei of mature cells (4, 10) has been seen in young plants only 5 mm long (11), but was not observed in zygotes fixed about 16 hours after fusion.

References

1. J. Parkinson, Theatrum Botanicum. London: Thos. Cotes, p. 1303 (1640).

2. J. Hämmerling, Ann. Rev. Plant Physiol. 14, 65 (1963).

3. C. J. Tandler, Naturwissenschaften 49, 112 (1962).

4. J.C.W. Crawley, Exp. Cell Res. 32, 368 (1963).

5. S. Granick, in The Cell (Eds. J. Bracket and A.E. Mirsky). New York: Academic Press, p. 489 (1961).

6. A. de Bary and E. Strassburger, Bot. Ztg. 35, 713 (1877).

7. L. G. Caro and R. P. van Tubergen, J. Cell Biol. 15, 173 (1962).

8. J.C.W. Crawley, Planta (Berl.) 69, 365 (1966).

9. J.C.W. Crawley, Z. miss. Mikrosk. 67, 136 (1966).

10. M. Bouloukhère. This symposium.

11. J.C.W. Crawley, Planta (Berl.) 65, 205 (1965).

Acknowledgements

The helpful advice of Professor Henry Harris, Dr T. Spencer and Mrs M. Coddington is gratefully acknowledged.

This work was carried out with the skilled assistance of Mr T. Cooper.

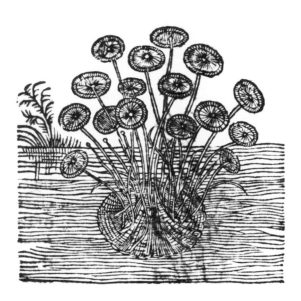

Fig. 1. Line drawing of Acetabularia mediterranea drawn by Parkinson in 1640 (ref. 1).

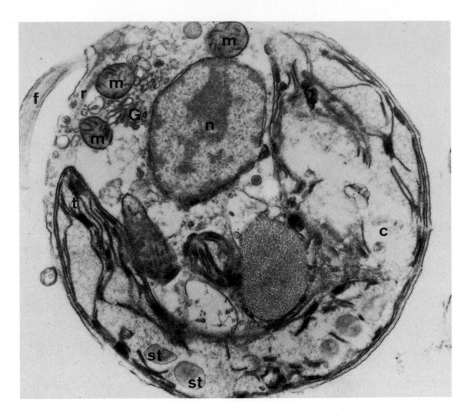

Fig. 2a. Section of a gamete x 22,000.
        f = flagellum; r = root of flagellum;
        n = nucleus; c = chloroplast;
        t = thylacoids; m = mitochondrion;
        st = starch grains; G = Golgi bodies.

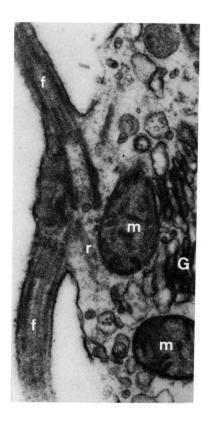

Fig. 2b. Nearby section x 45,000.

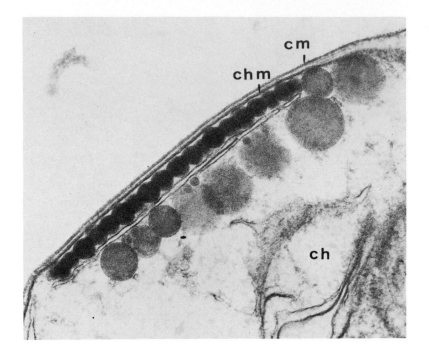

Fig. 3.   Eyespot in a gamete x 55,000
          cm = cell membrane
          chm = chloroplast membrane
          ch = chloroplast

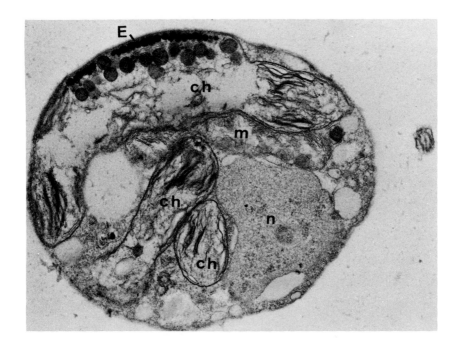

Fig. 4.   Section of a gamete x 18,000.
E = eyespot; ch = chloroplast;
n = nucleus; m = mitochondrion.

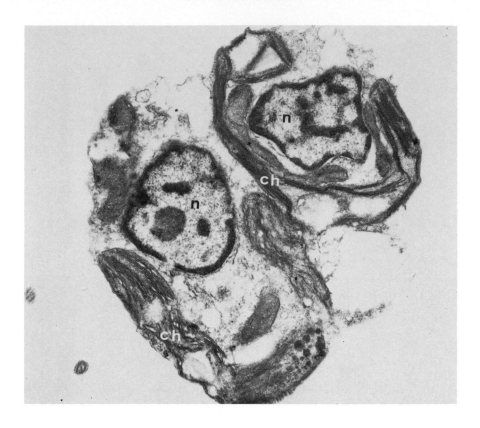

Fig. 5. Gametes just fusing x 18,000
         ch = chloroplast
         n = nucleus.

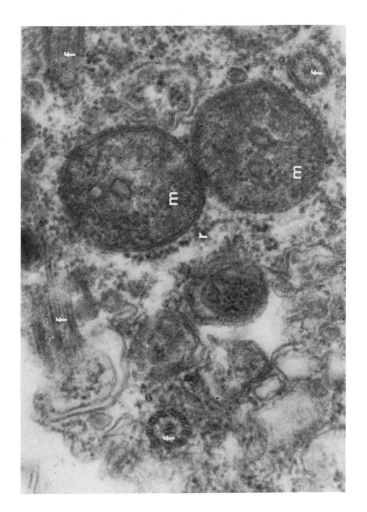

Fig. 6. Cytoplasm of fusing gametes x 50,000
f = flagellum; m = mitochondrion;
r = ribosomes.

JUNE 19 (RHODE-ST-GENÈSE)
MORNING SESSION

Chairman: Albert Jacques Bertinchamps

REGULATION OF ENZYME ACTIVITY DURING MORPHOGENESIS OF NUCLEATE AND ANUCLEATE CELLS OF ACETABULARIA

Klaus Zetsche, Gerd Ernst Grieninger, and Johannes Anders

Institut für Biologie der Universität Tübingen,
Germany.

Abstract

In Acetabularia mediterranea the activity of the UDPG-pyrophosphorylase is related to the development of the cap. The activity of the enzyme increases strongly when cap formation sets in. Similar changes in enzyme activity are observed in nucleate and anucleate cells. The activity of the Phosphoglucose-isomerase shows a different behaviour. The increase of activity of this enzyme follows the increase in total protein content. In addition to the correlation in time between cap formation and activity of the UDPG- pyrophosphorylase there exists a close correlation in space which is expressed in terms of a polar distribution of the enzyme.

In the unicellular green alga Acetabularia mediterranea the chemical composition of the polysaccharides which build up the cell wall of the stalk and of the cap or which may also be localized to some extent in the cytoplasm of this region differs. While the polysaccharides of the stalk and rhizoid region consist mainly of mannose and contain only minor amounts of glucose and galactose, the glucose and galactose content of the polysaccharides of the cap region is considerably greater. Rhamnose is found within the polysaccharides of the cap only. Furthermore the cell wall of the cysts which are formed in the mature cap after division of the primary nucleus and migration of the secondary nuclei into the cap is characterized by a relative high content of glucose and by a low content of mannose. In addition, the cyst wall contains minor amounts of galactose, rhamnose and xylose. By different extraction-techniques it was excluded that the high glucose content of the cyst wall results from starch contamination (Fig. 1).

In Acetabularia crenulata similar differences in the composition of the polysaccharides of the stalk and cap regions were found (Fig. 2; Zetsche 1967, Anders and Zetsche 1969).

It is well known that cells of Acetabularia from which the nucleus has been removed may still have considerable capacities of synthesis and morphogenesis. In addition to the formation of stalk and whorls of hairs, the morphogenetic capacities are expressed in the differentiation of the cap. It is very likely that these morphogenetic potentialities of anucleate cells are based on the presence of long-lived messenger RNA (Brachet et al. 1964; Brachet 1967; Hämmerling 1963; Zetsche, 1964, 1965, 1966 a and c).

Cells enucleated before initiation of cap formation also exhibit differences in the composition of the cell walls of stalk and of cap (Fig. 3). The processes which bring about differences in the composition of the polysaccharides of the stalk and cap region must therefore also take place within the enucleated cells (Zetsche 1967).

The question thus arises whether there are changes in the activity or in the synthesis of those enzymes which synthesize these sugars or incorporate them into the polysaccharides during the process of stalk, cap and cyst formation. It is known that during the synthesis of the polysaccharides nucleotide sugars play a decisive role as donors of sugar remnants which serve as building stones.

We looked therefore at the beginning of our present series of studies for enzymes which participate in the synthesis of nucleotide sugars. All the enzymes necessary for the synthesis of UDPG and of UDPGal from fructose-6-phosphate were shown to be present in A. mediterranea. We also found one GDPM-pyrophosphorylase (Zetsche 1966 b). Enzymes which synthesize Rhamnose and enzymes which incorporate sugars into the polysaccharides of the cell wall are being investigated at the present time (Fig. 4).

The activity of these enzymes during stalk and cap formation has been studied for UDPG-pyrophosphorylase, UDPG-4-epimerase and Phosphoglucose-isomerase, i.e. for those enzymes which catalyze the processes at the beginning and the end of the chain of synthesis (Zetsche 1966 d).

Since UDPG-4-epimerase shows generally the same characteristics as UDPG-pyrophosphorylase it suffices to consider this latter enzyme and the Phosphoglucose-isomerase. Let us consider first changes in activity of UDPG-pyrophosphorylase during morphogenesis of nucleate cells. As long as the plants form only stalk and whorls of hairs there is little increase in the activity of this enzyme. Activity increases greatly only when cap formation sets in. This increase is maintained as long as new caps are formed and cap growth takes place. The level of enzyme activity is maintained over a considerable period of time following completion of cap formation and growth. Since the rate of synthesis of proteins does not change during the transition from stalk to cap formation, the increase in the activity of the enzyme greatly surpasses the increase in total proteins (Fig. 5).

Similar changes in enzyme activity are observed in anucleate cells. As long as only stalk and whorls of hairs are formed, no or very little increase in enzyme activity takes place. Here, too, considerable increase in enzyme activity is found only during cap formation. Following completion of cap formation and growth the activity of the enzyme does not increase any further. The high level of activity is however again maintained over a considerable period of time (Fig. 6). The increase in enzyme activity is less in the anucleate plants than in the nucleate plants. This is to be expected since the percentage of cells which form caps is smaller in anucleate plants and, in addition, the caps formed are not as large. There exists therefore a close correlation in time between cap formation and increase in UDPG-pyrophosphorylase activity (Zetsche 1968).

In contrast to the behaviour of this enzyme the activity of the enzyme Phosphoglucose-isomerase increases to the same extent as the increase in total proteins (Fig. 7). The differences in behaviour of these enzymes during morphogenesis are demonstrated most clearly when they are examined in the same plants, as the results obtained with anucleate plants show (Fig. 8). It is evident that the

increase in the activity of the Phosphoglucose-isomerase
stops earlier than does the increase in the activity of
the UDPG-pyrophosphorylase (Grieninger 1969).

The question arises whether the increase in the activity of UDPG-pyrophosphorylase is based upon an increased synthesis of the enzyme at the time of cap formation
or merely upon the activation of enzyme molecules which
are already present. In order to answer this question
experiments were carried out in which plants were treated
with puromycin and actidione. Both antibiotics are known
to block the synthesis of proteins but the pathways
through which they act differ (Nathans 1964; Ellis 1969).

If these antibiotics are added to the culture medium of the plants shortly before initiation of cap formation the plants do not form caps and do not show any increase in enzyme activity. This inhibition is reversible.
When the plants are returned to a normal medium not containing these antibiotics a large number of them will form
caps after a while and the cap formation is accompanied
by a great increase in enzyme activity. Results obtained
with nucleate and anucleate cells are basically the same
(Fig. 9). It is most likely therefore that the increase
in the activity of UDPG-pyrophosphorylase during cap formation is based upon increased synthesis of the enzyme
(Zetsche 1968).

Since this increase in the synthesis of the enzyme
also takes place within anucleate cells, the regulation
of the synthesis of the UDPG-pyrophosphorylase must take
place within the cytoplasm. One may think here primarily
of two possibilities:
1. Regulation takes place at the level of translation.
2. Genes responsible for the synthesis of the enzymes
are present within extranuclear DNA, in particular DNA
within chloroplasts. In this case increase in the synthesis of the enzyme could be brought about through activation of these extranuclear genes. However, the experiments
described below largely exclude this second possibility.

When nucleate posterior pieces of stalk which do
not contain a storage of carriers of information are treated with 10 µg/ml of actinomycin the synthesis of UDPG-
pyrophosphorylase is almost completely blocked (Fig. 10).
On the other hand the same concentration of actinomycin
has no influence on the increase in enzyme activity in
anucleate cells which contain a storage of long-lived

messenger RNA within the tip region of the stalk (Fig.11).
It may be objected that actinomycin cannot block chloroplast DNA for reasons of permeability, etc. Since however
actinomycin strongly inhibits incease in chlorophyll within anucleate cells this objection is not supported. In addition, we were able to show that although chloramphenicol
(100 µg/ml) almost completely blocks increase in chlorophyll both in nucleate and in anucleate cells, it inhibits initially the synthesis of UDPG-pyrophosphorylase
only very little (nucleate posterior pieces of stalk) or
not at all (anucleate cells). Inhibition which sets in
later is very likely a secondary effect based upon a
strong decrease in the capacity of treated cells to photo-
synthesize (Zetsche 1969).

It is known that chloramphenicol inhibits specifically the protein synthesis at the site of the 70 S -ri-
bosomes (Ellis 1969). One may conclude therefore that the
synthesis of the UDPG-pyrophosphorylase does not take
place at the site of the 70 S -ribosomes of the chloroplasts but rather at the site of the 80 S -ribosomes of
the cytoplasm. Thus the possibility of the regulation of
the synthesis of UDPG-pyrophosphorylase through activation of extranuclear genes is largely excluded and all
results support a system of regulation at the level of
translation.

We assume that a large portion of the UDPG-pyrophosphorylase messenger RNA is formed through nuclear
genes long before cap formation and is stored within the
cytoplasm in its non-active form. Activation of this
type of messenger RNA takes place only at the beginning
of cap formation. How is the time of activation determined ? The following results may help to clarify this
point.

Cells which already contain within their cytoplasm the messenger RNA necessary for cap formation form
caps earlier if one removes the nucleus by cutting off the
rhizoid or blocks it by addition of actinomycin (Beth
1953; Zetsche 1966 e). The nucleus has inhibitory effects
upon the realization of the information about cap formation within the cytoplasm, possibly by means of substances which suppress the translation of the respective messenger RNA.

The close connection between cap formation and
increase in the synthesis of UDPG-pyrophosphorylase can

91

be made to disappear through treatment of plants with p-fluorophenylalanine. As we already observed, this compound specifically inhibits cap formation in A. mediterranea while stalk formation and the synthesis of proteins is influenced little or not at all (Zetsche 1966 c). It is evident from Figure 12 that p-fluorophenylalanine has no influence on the normal change in activity of UDPG-pyrophosphorylase in nucleate cells although it strongly inhibits cap formation. The increase in enzyme activity sets in within treated cells at the same time as in untreated cells, i.e. at the time when cap formation would normally have taken place (Zetsche 1969).

We interpret these results to mean that increased synthesis of the UDPG-pyrophosphorylase is only one of many processes which are necessary in order to initiate formation of caps. Once these processes have begun apparently proceed automatically independent of whether cap formation takes place or not.

In addition to the correlation in time between cap formation and activity of the UDPG-pyrophosphorylase there exists a close correlation in space which is expressed in terms of a polar distribution of the enzyme.

Cells not containing caps are cut into three pieces of equal length, i.e. an apical, a middle, and a basal piece. The activity of the UDPG-pyrophosphorylase is examined for each piece and the activity is related to 10 µg-protein-N. The protein content of the various pieces is approximately the same but the enzyme activity shows great differences. The activity of the enzyme is highest in the apical piece, while toward the basal end it decreases sharply (Fig. 13). Thus even before cap formation there exists an apico-basal gradient of enzyme activity. This gradient appears to be related to the predominant synthesis of the cell wall at the tip region of the stalk.

The same experiment was carried out with cells which had already formed a small cap. Enzyme activity again showed a strong apico-basal gradient (Fig. 14). There are considerable differences in the absolute values of enzyme activity between cells of different cultures, but all cells show this apico-basal gradient of enzyme activity.

What causes this unequal distribution of enzyme activity within the cell ? Is it due to differences in the distribution of enzyme inhibitors or enzyme destruction during preparation ?   The following experiments were carried out in order to answer these questions.

Series of dilutions were prepared from the homogenate of the apical and middle pieces. There is an exact linear relationship between the amount of homogenate used and enzyme activity. In addition, homogenates of apical and of basal pieces were dialyzed over night against a buffer. The same differences in activity were found between the dialyzed homogenates as were found to exist before dialysis. These results indicate that no activators or inhibitors are present. Finally apical and basal pieces were homogenized both separately and together. Enzyme activity then showed only additive behaviour. This latter result excludes the possibility of differential inactivation of the enzyme during its preparation. We conclude therefore that the differences in activity between different regions of the cell are based upon differences in the amount of enzyme present within these regions. There are in particular two possible explanations for the polar distribution of the enzyme:
1.   The enzyme is synthesized from the beginning in greater amounts in the apical than in the basal regions of the cell.
2.   The enzyme is synthesized evenly throughout the cell but subsequently there is a preferential transport into the tip region of the stalk resulting in an accumulation of the enzyme within this region.

In order to answer these questions enzyme activity of the segments was determined not only immediately following isolation of the segments through cutting but also after the isolated segments had been left to grow for a further 31 days. As has already been mentioned, a level of activity is reached at this time which is maintained over a considerable period. The apical and middle pieces examined show approximately the same amount of growth in terms of stalk length, but the basal pieces exhibit much less morphogenetic capacity (Fig. 15 and 16). Only apical pieces are able to differentiate caps, and each apical piece shows cap formation. At the time of isolation the protein content of the three types of segments is approximately the same. In the following period of growth the different types of segment then show progressively greater differences in their capacity to synthesize proteins : the basal segments form only half the

93

amount of protein formed by the apical and the middle pieces. The enzyme activity per segment immediately following isolation of the segment is highest within the apical segment and lowest within the basal segment. This is true even though the activity of the enzyme is related to protein nitrogen.

During culture of the isolated segments for 31 days the enzyme activity per segment increases most sharply in the apical segments. Increase in enzyme activity is less within the middle and least in the basal segments. Since the increase in enzyme activity in the apical segments greatly exceeds the increase in protein, we also find a greater specific enzyme activity in the apical segment on the 31st day of culture. Observation of the changes in activity with time indicates that the rates of increase in activity do not differ initially very much between the three types of segment. Significant differences are not apparent until the 16th day after isolation. Enzyme activity now increases sharply in the apical pieces but only slightly in the middle and basal segments (Fig. 17).

These results demonstrate clearly that the polar distribution of the enzyme is the result of a preferential synthesis of the enzyme in the apical region of the stalk. The rate of enzyme synthesis is higher within the apical piece than in the middle and basal segments, and this is particularly evident at the time of onset of cap formation (Zetsche 1969).

What mechanism determines the varying capacities of the apical, middle and basal segments to synthesize the enzyme ?   One may propose in particular two hypotheses:

1.The messenger RNA responsible for the synthesis of UDPG-pyrophosphorylase is distributed in form of an apico-basal concentration gradient. This corresponds to the concept of distribution of "morphogenetic substances" proposed by Hämmerling for <u>Acetabularia</u> (Hämmerling 1934).

2.The messenger RNA is evenly distributed throughout the cell but for reasons not yet known translation of the messenger RNA mainly takes place in the apical region of the cell.

The first-mentioned hypothesis is supported by results obtained by Hämmerling (1934) in his experiments on regeneration and transplantation. These indicate the existence of an apico-basal gradient in the distribution of the morphogenetic substances responsible for stalk, whorl and cap formation. It is very likely that these morphogenetic substances are indentical with messenger RNA which specifies the synthesis of the enzymes necessary for morphogenesis.

If we accept an apico-basal gradient in the concentration of the messenger RNA responsible for the UDPG- -pyrophosphorylase then this implies that the messenger RNA which is synthesized within the nucleus in the rhizoidal end of the cell must be transported over a distance of 60 mm in a polar direction toward the tip of the stalk and accumulated here. Unequal distribution of messenger RNA may thus represent an important factor in the morphogenesis of the cell. However, it remains to be shown how such a distribution is brought about.

Acknowledgements

We wish to thank Prof. K. v. Maltzahn for the translation of the manuscript.

References

Anders, J. and K. Zetsche : unpublished work.
Beth, K.: Z. Naturforsch. 8 b, 771 (1953).
Brachet, J. ; H. Denis and F. De Vitry :
Develop. Biol. 9, 398 (1964).
Brachet, J.: Nature 213, 650 (1967).
Ellis, R.: Science 163, 477 (1969).
Grieninger, G. : unpublished work.
Hämmerling, J.: Arch. Entwicklungsmech. Organ. 131, 1
               (1934).
            - Ann. Rev. Plant Physiol. 14, 65 (1963).
Nathans, D.: Proc. nat. Acad. Sci. (Wash.) 51, 585
               (1964).
Zetsche, K. : Z. Naturforsch. 19 b, 751 (1964).
            - Planta 64, 119 (1965).
            - Z. Naturforsch. 21 b, 88 (1966 a).
            - Planta 68, 240 (1966 b).
            - Planta 68, 360 (1966 c).

- Biochim. biophys. Acta (Amst.) 124, 332 (1966 d).
- Z. Naturforsch. 21 b, 375 (1966 e).
- Planta 76, 326 (1967).
- Z. Naturforsch. 23 b, 369 (1968).
- Planta in press (1969).
- unpublished work.

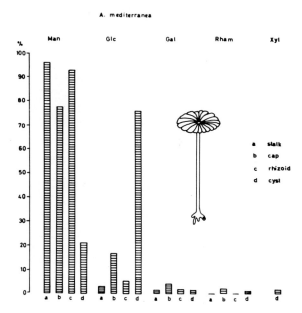

Fig. 1 : Composition of the polysaccharides present in different cell regions of Acetabularia mediterranea.
Ordinate = sugars in per cent of total neutral sugars.

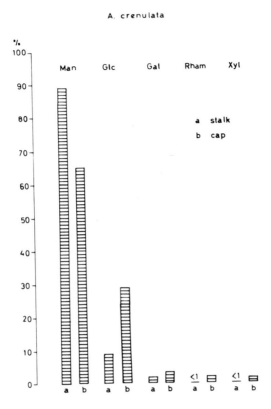

Fig. 2 :   Composition of the polysaccharides present in
different regions of Acetabularia crenulata.
Ordinate = sugars in per cent of total neutral
sugars.

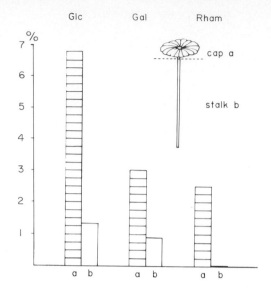

Fig. 3 : Composition of the polysaccharides of the stalk
and cap region of <u>A. mediterranea</u>. Cells enucleated prior to cap formation.
Ordinate = sugars in per cent of cell wall dry
weights.

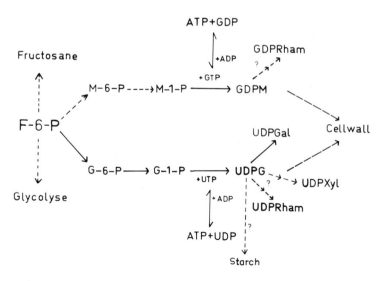

Fig. 4 : Enzymes of sugar metabolism in <u>A. mediterranea</u>.
Unbroken arrows: enzymes demonstrated
Broken arrows: enzymes so far not detected

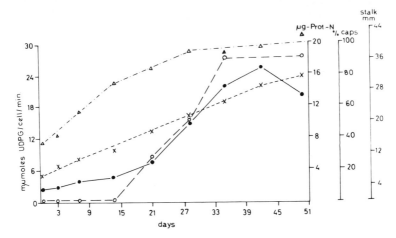

Fig. 5 : Activity of UDPG-pyrophosphorylase in nucleate
cells.
●——● enzyme activity; o— — o cap formation;
✕---✕ protein-N/cell; △--·--△ stalk length/cell;

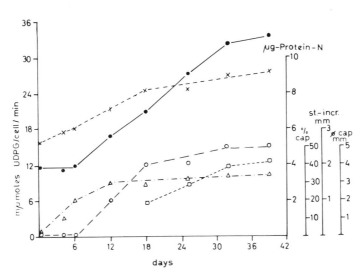

Fig. 6 : Activity of UDPG-pyrophosphorylase in enucleated
cells.
●——● enzyme activity; o— — —o cells with cap;
✕---✕protein-N/cell; △--·--△ increase of
stalk length/cell; ☐---☐diameter of the caps.

99

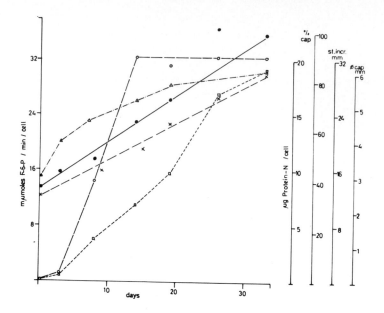

Fig. 7 : Activity of Phosphoglucose-isomerase in nucleate
cells;
 ●——● activity of Phosphoglucose-isomerase;
✕--✕μg protein-N/cell; △·—·—△ stalk increa-
se/cell; ○——○ plants with cap; ☐----☐
diameter of the caps.

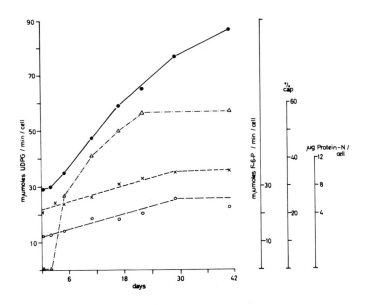

Fig. 8 : Activity of Phosphoglucose-isomerase and activity
of UDPG-pyrophosphorylase in enucleated cells.
●——● activity of UDPG-pyrophosphorylase;
✕- -✕µg protein-N/cell; o - - - -o activity
of Phosphoglucose-isomerase; △·—·△ plants
with cap.

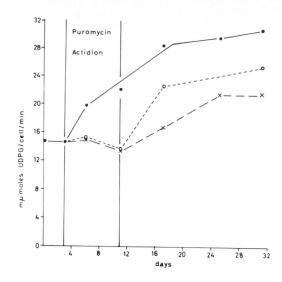

Fig. 9 :   Effect of puromycin and actidione on the activity of UDPG-pyrophosphorylase in enucleated
cells.

●———● control cells; o----o cells treated
with puromycin (30 µg/ml);✗---✗ cells treated
with actidione (0,25 µg/ml).
The antibiotics were added three days after
enucleation. On the 11th day the cells were transferred to a culture medium free of antibiotics.

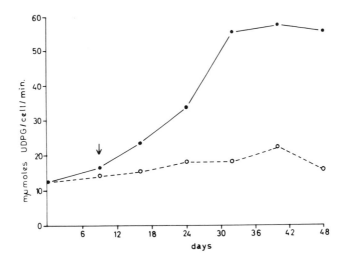

Fig.10 : Effect of actinomycin on the activity of UDPG-
-pyrophosphorylase in nucleate posterior parts
of the cell.
●———● control cells; o – – – o cells treated
with actinomycin;   ↓   initiation of cap formation in the control cells.

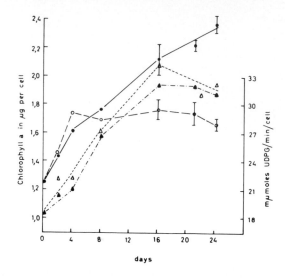

Fig. 11 : Effect of actinomycin on the activity of UDPG-
-pyrophosphorylase and on the content of chlorophyll a of enucleated cells.
▲·—·-▲ enzyme activity of control cells;
△----△ enzyme activity of cells treated with
actinomycin (10 μg/ml); ●———● chlorophyll a
content of control cells; o—— o chlorophyll a
content of cells treated with actinomycin. No
lag phase in increase of enzyme activity occurs
because cap initiation starts immediately after
enucleation.

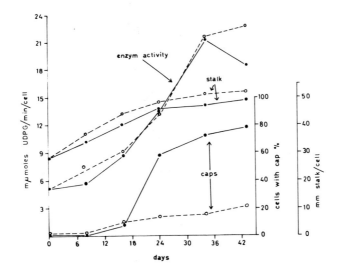

Fig.12 : Effect of p-fluorophenylalanine on the activity
of UDPG-pyrophosphorylase in nucleate cells.
●———● control cells; o----o cells treated
with p-fluorophenylalanine.

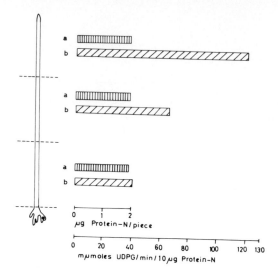

Fig.13 : Activity of UDPG-pyrophosphorylase in different cell regions.
a) protein-N/piece; b) enzyme activity/10 µg protein-N.

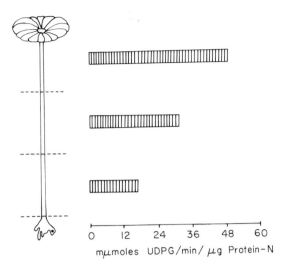

Fig.14 : Activity of UDPG-pyrophosphorylase in different cell regions of cells with caps.

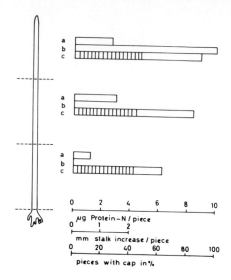

Fig. 15 : The morphogenetic and protein synthesizing capacities of different cell pieces (initial
length 15 mm).
a) stalk increase;
b) pieces with cap at day 31;
c) column with hatching: protein-N at day 0,
blank column: protein-N at day 31.

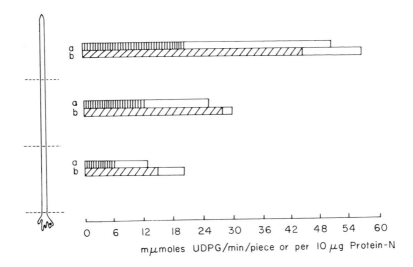

Fig. 16 : Activity of UDPG-pyrophosphorylase in different cell pieces (the same material as described in Fig. 15) after culturing for 31 days.
a) column with hatching: enzyme activity/piece
at day 0, blank column: increase of enzyme ac-
tivity/piece up to day 31;
b) the same as in a)
but enzyme activity per 10 µg-protein-N.

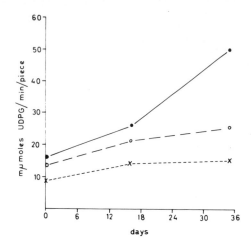

Fig. 17 : Changes of UDPG-pyrophosphorylase activity in
different cell pieces with time.
●——● apical pieces; o — — -o middle pieces;
X- - -X basal pieces.

PLASTID STRUCTURE AND THE EVOLUTION
OF PLASTIDS IN ACETABULARIA

Simone Puiseux-Dao and Anne-Catherine Dazy

Laboratoire de Biologie Cellulaire Végétale
1 rue M. Arnoux, 92-Montrouge, France

Abstract

An analysis of plastid structure in Acetabularia is
reported with an interpretation scheme for plastidal division. The plastidal population presents a rhythmic evolution due to the replication of basic structural units and
to the separation of the linked units ; such an evolution
gives an exponential growth to this plastidal population.
The plastid division is controlled by a nuclear substance
distributed in an apicobasal fashion in the cytoplasm.

Interrelations between the cell nucleus and organelles containing satellite DNA may be studied with certain
convenient materials. One such material is the unicellular
alga Acetabularia mediterranea whose giant cell possesses
a single nucleus and numerous plastids and mitochondria.
The ovoid chloroplasts measure 3-8 μ long by 1-3 μ wide and
are sufficiently large to be observed with the light microscope. Their longitudinal axes are disposed more or less
parallel to the longitudinal axis of the cylindrical cell.
In certain respects, their aspect changes during culture.
During the 12 hours photoperiod, these changes follow a
pattern which may be related to the evolution of the plastid population of the cell.

1. The structure and division of the plastids.

With the culture conditions used which favour poly-saccharide synthesis (t°:24-27°C ; light: 3000 lux ; 12h Light-12 h Dark), the upper of the algae (Acetabularia: 2 to 4 cm long) contained chloroplasts which appeared as green rods containing 1, 2 or 3 (sometimes more) polysac-charide grains. In the midregion, many plastids appeared rounded due to an increase in the size of the polysaccha-ride grains. In the basal part of the cell, chloroplasts were often very large and filled with polysaccharides. Thus, the cells contained both "long" and "globular" chlo-roplasts with the globular forms corresponding to trans-formed rods. These two classes of chloroplasts observed with the light microscope were distributed along two oppo-site apicobasal gradients.

The ultrastructure of the "long" Acetabularia chlo-roplasts is very simple. They are surrounded by an exter-nal double membrane with peripheral lamellae and polysac-charide grains inside (Fig.1). DNA fibers are observed be-tween the grains and the most internal lamellae. Ribosomes and lipid droplets are scattered in the stroma. The geome-try of the lamellae is best studied using longitudinal axial section of plastids. In those which contain one gra-nule, the lamellae are disposed in two groups symetrical with respect to a near axial plane. This peculiar dispo-sition of lamellae allows us to recognize two opposite poles in each chloroplast. When isolated, these thylacoids appear as long plied ribbons partly stuck together by the edge. Sometimes the internal thylacoids appear broader than the external thylacoids. When chloroplasts contain two po-lysaccharide grains, they also possess two peripheral groups of lamellae but some diagonal thylacoids diverge from the poles to separate the two grains. With such a pattern, each half chloroplast has the same structure as a one-grain plastid since each of the two grains is sur-rounded by lamellae. Thus, the 2-grain chloroplast can be considered as composed of two similar plastidal units (Fig.1). In the long chloroplasts with 3, 4 or more poly-saccharide grains, diagonal lamellae always exist between the grains and these plastids are considered to be compo-sed of 3, 4 or more units. A similar interpretation appears to be applicable to the round chloroplasts, but the arran-gements is less regular due to the large size of the polysaccharide grains. The thylacoids of the round chloroplasts are not very well developed which is suggestive of an inhibition of thylacoid synthesis when the contents of carbohydrate reserves reach a high level. Many figures have been observed with the electron microscope that suggest the separation of one plastidal unit from another (fission). The process is easiest to visualize with two-grain plastids. Here the peripheral lamellae seem to separate followed by separation of the two granules, each surrounded by their own thylacoids (Fig.1). Finally, separation and repair of the plastid envelope would result in the formation of two daughter chloroplasts. New polysaccharide centers seem to arise amid the lamellae beneath or opposite the point of envelope rupture and repair.

Thus, Acetabularia chloroplasts can be considered as consisting of multiple units with each unit containing at least three kinds of membranes : envelope, peripheral lamellae and diagonal lamellae. Some evidence suggests different functions for the two kinds of lamellae. Algae cultured in darkness have very large plastids and certain figures observed with the electron microscope can be explained by fusion of normal chloroplasts. In such long plastids and with our culture conditions, polysaccharide grains are visible after several weeks in darkness, the envelope is well defined, diagonal lamellae are present but the peripheral thylacoids appear as piles of numerous short discs. These observations suggest that the peripheral thylacoids whose aspect is disturbed by darkness, are especially concerned with photosynthesis. The diagonal lamellae might be involved with DNA replication or separation since DNA is always in contact with their internal surface. A diagram consistent with the images observed is presented to summarize our concepts of plastid division (Fig. 2).

II. The plastidal population in Acetabularia cells.

Additional information supporting the concept of a plastidal unit in Acetabularia came from studies which showed that the number of polysaccharide grains per plastid followed a regular pattern of cyclic change during a 12 hour photoperiod. Cells were fixed with glutaraldehyde,

washed with buffer and stained with Lugol solution for
light microscope examination. Parallel counts were made
with the electron microscope on longitudinal serial
sections. Material was fixed at intervals of 1 hour from
9:00 a.m. to 7:00 p.m. during the 12 hour photoperiod.
At the beginning of the photoperiod, 1- and 2- unit plastids prevailed in the upper part of the algae while 3
(or more)-unit plastids were rare. Progressively during
the next 10 hours, the number of 1-unit plastids decreased and 3 (or more)-unit chloroplasts became more numerous. Then about 5:00 p.m., the situation reversed with
the number of 1-unit plastids increasing again. This pe-
riodic evolution of different plastid forms would seem to
support the plastidal unit concept. The situation rever-
ses upon the separation of units at the end of the afternoon (Fig.3). We calculate (Puiseux-Dao, 1968) that such
an evolution gives an exponential growth for the plastid
population consistent with the data of Shephard (sp.)
(1965).

The above observation concerns only the chloroplasts of the upper and middle parts of the cells. More
than the population of the round plastids in the basal
part is always composed of 2 and more unit plastids even
early in the morning. Here, the dividing process seems to
be slower as growth of lamellae, even diagonal ones, is
restricted. So it is possible to think that polysaccharide
deposition in Acetabularia chloroplasts prevails when division and lamellae synthesis decrease; a kind of feed-
back regulation should occur. It can be supposed too that
DNA synthesis is also included in this regulation process;
effectively, DNA regions are encountered in these basal
round plastids with less frequency than in the chloroplasts
of the upper portions of the algae. These findings agree
with those of Woodcock and Bogorad (1968) who showed that
the quantity of DNA in Acetabularia plastids varies, ap-
proaching zero for some.

The two opposite gradients for distribution of long
and round plastids may be linked to their ability to divide. As the gradient concerning long dividing chloroplasts shows a localization similar to that of "nuclear
morphogenetic substances" in Acetabularia, a simple hypothesis is that plastid division is controlled by nuclear
substances distributed in an apicobasal fashion in the

114

cytoplasm. To test the hypothesis of a gradient of nuclear
morphogenetic substances affecting chloroplast division,
we studied chloroplasts in regenerating short basal parts
where a new apicobasal gradient of nuclear substances is
elaborated. After two days following decapitation, the
plastid population was changed. The polysaccharide grains
of the plastids were small in the upper part of the regenerating cells and could not be detected in the developing
apex. Counting units in chloroplasts just beneath the apex,
showed that 1-unit plastids prevailed in the morning as in
the upper part of normal cells. This distribution confor-
med to the region where new nuclear substances were accu-
mulating. Besides with cut algae placed in culture medium
containing ribonuclease (1 mg/ml) which inhibits regeneration in Acetabularia, the following results were observed. After 48 h treatment, the plants could be separated
into 3 groups : in the first, the cells did not grow at
all, in the second, a few algae seem to grow a little, in
the third, new short apices about 1 mm long could be seen.
So the inhibition of regeneration by ribonuclease does not
occur immediately.Then in the 3 batches of plants, plastids
with 1, 2 or more grains were counted in the apical parts
and a good correlation between the growth capacity and the
aspect of the plastid population is to be reported ; in
non regenerating algae, the chloroplasts in the apice look
like those of Acetabularia basal parts, in regenerating
algae, the plastid population in the apice is similar to
that of a normal Acetabularia apical part (Fig.4). Such
observations seem to support the above hypothesis. However,
the replicating ability of chloroplasts, controlled by
nuclear substances distributed with an apicobasal gradient
in the cytoplasm, should give a perfectly regular distribution of light and rounder plastids along the axis of the
cell, instead of the two apparent observed gradients. In
fact, cytoplasmic streaming currents transport the long
light chloroplasts but not the heavy round ones which mix
the plastids somewhat. But the apicobasal gradient of
plastid distribution ends to be preserved, because long
chloroplasts placed in the basal part of the algae must
more or less rapidly be transformed into round ones because of the absence of nuclear active substances controlling plastidal replication.

Ethidium bromide (BET) which is known to inhibit

mitochondrial DNA synthesis, was used in some experiments
in order to study its effects on plastids. It was added
to the culture media of Acetabularia cells (20 to 120
µg/ml - 2 to 7 days); because of the drug's orange red
colour in solution, controls were cultivated under filters made with the solutions themselves. Morphological
anomalies were observed in the treated plants. Counts of
plastids (Fig.3) with 1, 2, 3 or more grains made at
different times during the light period show that in the
controls more replicating chloroplasts are situated in
the middle of the axis; the simplest explanation would be
suppose that orange red light inhibits the transport of
nuclear substances in the cytoplasm but does not inhibit
their activation. In the BET treated algae the rhythm of
the chloroplast multiplication disappears; studies of
the curves obtained suggest that the separation of pre-
existing plastid units goes on slowly but that initiation
of new units is completely arrested which could be predic-
ted if BET stops DNA synthesis in these organelles (Dazy,
in preparation).

New experiments are initiated in the hope of adding
new arguments to our hypothesis on the structure, function and nuclear control of plastidal units in Acetabularia.

Acknowledgements

We wish to thank Professor Morré for the translation of the manuscript.

References

- S. Puiseux-Dao, C.R. Acad. Sci. 256, 1382–1384 (1968).
- D. Shephard, Exptl Cell Res. 37, 93–110 (1965).
- C.L. Woodcock and L. Bogorad, 8th Ann. Meeting of the Ann. Soc. for Cell Biol. (1968).

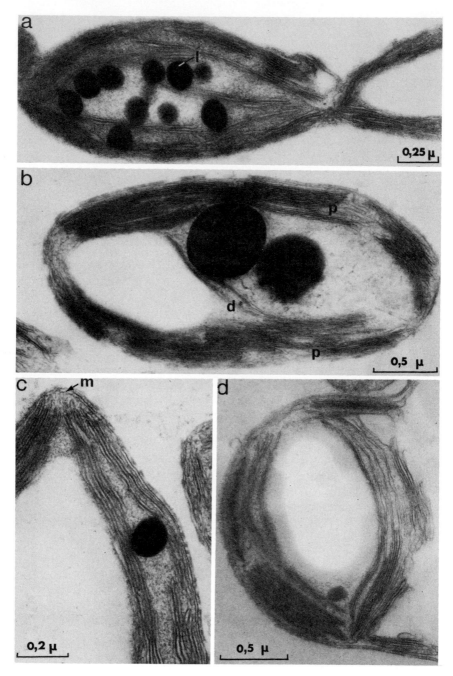

Fig.1 a: <u>Acetabularia mediterranea</u> plastid in tangential longitudinal section; groups of lamellae are visible in the stroma which contains lipid droplets (1).

b: a two-unit plastid observed in an alga kept in darkness during two weeks and illuminated again 15 minutes. Numerous lamellae are disposed peripherally (p), diagonal lamellae are seen between one polysaccharide grain cut in the plan of section and a stroma region which surrounds another grain.

c: a chloroplast's pole which shows the external membrane (m) and the two groups of diverging lamellae.

d: a plastidal unit separating from a plastid (same conditions as b).

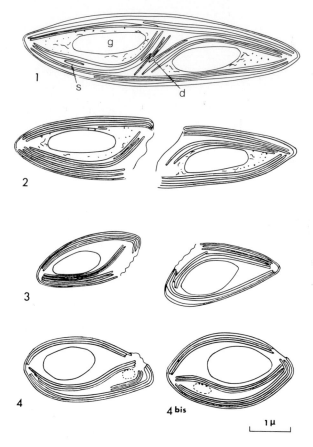

Fig.2 : The division of plastids in <u>Acetabularia</u> : a schematic representation. 1, 2, 3: successive stages of the division ; 4 : formation of a new polysaccharide center.

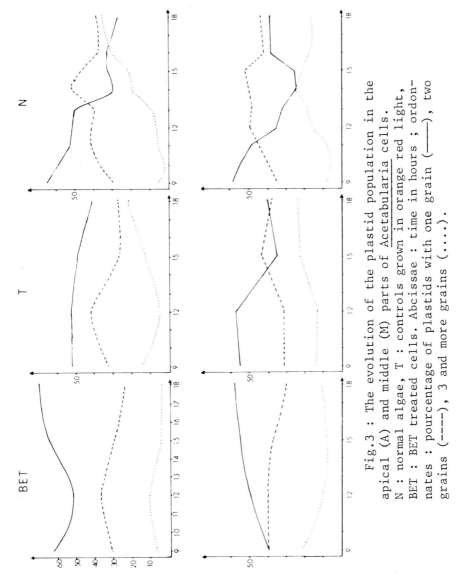

Fig.3 : The evolution of the plastid population in the apical (A) and middle (M) parts of Acetabularia cells. N : normal algae, T : controls grown in orange red light, BET : BET treated cells. Abcissae : time in hours ; ordonnates : pourcentage of plastids with one grain (——), two grains (----), 3 and more grains (....).

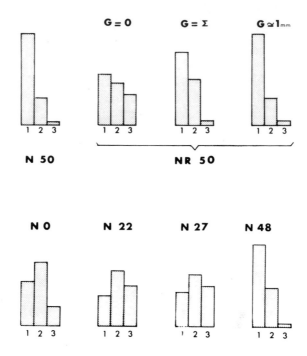

Fig.4 : Aspects of plastid population in regenerating
Acetabularia basal parts. 1 : NO: pourcentage of plastids
with one grain (1), 2 grains (2), 3 grains and more (3)
just before cutting at 10 a.m. N22. The same 22 hours later,
N27: 27 hours later ; N48: 48 hours later. 2 : N50 : pourcentage of plastids 50 hours after cutting. NR50 : the same
in regenerating algae treated by RNAase which can be distributed in three groups. G = o : no regenerating algae ;
G = ε : algae with a very short new apex; G ∿ 1 mm : algae
with an apical point about 1 mm long.

AFTERNOON SESSION

Chairman: Maurice Errera

MECHANISMS IN CELL WALL FORMATION IN ACETABULARIA

Günther Werz

Max- Plank- Institut für Zellbiologie,
Wilhelmshaven, Germany.

Abstract

The shape of species-specific characteristics of
a plant cell, like Acetabularia, is determined by the morphogenesis of the cytoplasm and not by the mode of the
cell wall's growth. In the course of cytoplasm- morphogenesis the peripheral regions of the plasm acquire specific structural and functional properties, by which they
become qualified for cell wall formation, and for controlling cell wall quality. These morphogenetic events are
nucleus- dependent, but are regulated by certain cytoplasmic mechanisms.

Introduction

Species-specific differences between plant cells
are principally revealed by the different appearances of
the cell wall architectures. The mechanisms of cell wall
formation in plant cells are, therefore, important parts
of cell morphogenesis. Heslop- Harrison (1968) mentioned
that "... the modes of growth of the wall determine cell
shape..." (see also Nickerson 1964; Hämmerling and Zetsche
1966). This statement implies a control of the species-
specificity of the cell's morphology by the cell wall
formation processes, and logically includes their involvement in directing cell morphogenesis. But as it stands now,
another aspect should also be considered with regard to

morphogenesis : the determination of the species- specific morphological appearances of cells by cytoplasm- morphogenesis, which not only leads to the plasmatic model of species characteristics, but rather directs specificity of cell wall formation.

Detailed consideration of cytoplasm-morphogenesis in plant cells is only rarely found in the literature (see Bloch 1965; Roelofsen 1965). This probably depends on the fact that cell wall formation unquestionably bases on specific cytoplasmic functions. Thus cellular morphogenesis cannot easily be dissociated into processes of cytoplasmic morphogenesis and the formation of the corresponding cell walls. Both processes are closely related, and each one is highly complex in nature. Moreover, they normally take place within very narrow time limits and are regulated in such a way that cell wall formation is the terminal link in the chain of morphogenetic events.

One exception are certain morphogenetic processes in the unicellular and uninucleate green algae Acetabularia. This object is not only suitable for detail-studies of morphogenesis, but also proved to be an excellent model for observing and experimentally inducing dissociation of cytoplasm- morphogenesis and cell wall formation. In the following, therefore, experimental evidences for this basic morphogenetic principle operating in the Acetabularia cells will be presented. Furthermore, results concerning the functions in inducing and controlling species- specific cell wall formation of distinctly structured marginal regions of the cytoplasm will be discussed.

Cytoplasm- morphogenesis,
basic determinant of cell wall specificity

The vegetative phases of the development of an Acetabularia cell are terminated by the disintegration of the giant primary nucleus, which normally is located within the rhizoid (fig.1). The disintegration is induced by non- specific cytoplasmic mechanisms (Hämmerling 1939; Werz, unpubl.) , and gives rise to small secondary nuclei, which multiply rapidly by mitoses (see Schulze 1939). At least these nuclei migrate through the stalk into the cap rays, where they initiate a special morphogenetic process: the formation of cysts (fig. 2).

Investigations on details of this specific process led to the following results. The cytoplasm of the cap rays is unable to form cysts. Only under the influences of the secondary nuclei the cytoplasmic layer of the cap rays is partitioned into circumscribed portions of cyto- plasm, each of which contains one nucleus (fig. 2 a,b). This plasma- partition is followed by growth of the cyto- plasm towards the cap ray's center, and finally is com- pleted by separation of the pear- shaped compartments from each other (fig. 2 c,d). By contraction of the cytoplasmic compartments the definite species- specific cytoplasmic model of the cysts is formed (fig. 2 e). They are delimited by a plasma membrane (fig. 3), but a cell wall is not present at this time. Cyst specific cell wall formation is induced only after the cytoplasmic mor- phogenesis of the cysts is terminated (fig. 2 f). Accor- ding to its fine structural features the cyst wall of Ace- tabularia cells gives a color reaction with chlor- zink- iodine- reagent, which is usually used for the demonstra- tion of cellulose. In this context, however, it should be added that the cyst wall is not pure cellulose, but is mainly composed of galactose, glucose, mannose, and xylose (Werz 1968 a,b; 1969 a,b).

Cyst formation is a relatively simple morphogenetic process. But nevertheless it clearly shows that it is not the mode of growth of the cell wall that determines the morphology of the cell's shape. It rather shows that the preceding nucleus- dependent cytoplasmic morphogenesis determines the shape of species- characteristics and the quality of their cell walls.

This conclusion implies that the formation of an abnormal cytoplasmic model should result in an abnormal shape of the cell's wall, while the composition and the fine structural features of the cell wall should be nor- mal. This hypothesis was examined experimentally : when Actinomycin- D or Puromycin is applicated for short times to the early stages of cyst development, or when the cells are treated with higher than optimal temperatures for some time, abnormal cysts are formed (Werz 1968 a). In accor- dance with the hypothesis such "cysts" base on abnormal plasmatic cyst models. In spite of the abnormal shape, however, the cell wall which is synthesized on the abnormal cyst model exhibits normal chemical and fine structural properties.

The problem "morphogenesis" of a plant cell is, therefore, not primarily a question of the mechanisms of the cell wall's growth, but rather is the question of the mechanisms, which cause the cytoplasm to differentiate specific functional features, which cause induction of cell wall formation and control its specificity.

The experiments from which these conclusions were drawn, were concerned with cyst development in situ. Under these conditions, however, the possibility cannot be excluded that the differentiation process is stimulated and (or) is regulated by components of the pre- existing cell wall. One might think of the possibility that such components influence the specific compartition processes of the cytoplasm, and thus are controlling cell wall formation processes. In order to examine this question living "undifferentiated" cytoplasm was isolated from the cap rays, and was maintained in vitro.

Figure 4 shows the morphogenetic behaviour of isolated nucleate cytoplasm. These "protoplasts" are consistently able to form "cysts", and to initiate specific cyst wall synthesis (fig. 4 d).

The capabilities of anucleate isolated cytoplasm, according to Gibor (1965) called "cytoplasts", are quite different (fig. 5). Cytoplasts of cap ray plasm which not yet had contained a nucleus are neither able to form a cytoplasmic cyst model, nor are they able to synthesize cyst wall, a behaviour that clearly shows that the cytoplasm was not able to undergo those differentiation processes which lead to its special functional properties. If, however, a nucleus had been allowed to function within the cap ray plasm for some time and was then removed, also cytoplasts have received a certain degree of differentiation capability, by which they became able of synthesizing a limited amount of cyst wall.

These results, obtained with cytoplasm in vitro are in agreement with those obtained with the cytoplasm in situ. They give further evidence that cell wall formation is governed by the nucleus at the base. They show, however, that initiation of cell wall synthesis does not require the presence of the nucleus, but is dependent on cytoplasmic functions. We may, therefore, conclude, that specific information had been transferred from the nucleus into the cytoplasm, where it is converted into special functional properties, also when the nucleus is removed (see Werz 1968 a,b).

Structural properties of the cytoplasm, and their relation to cell wall formation

It has been demonstrated that morphogenesis of the cytoplasm is connected with the development of special functional properties in peripheral cytoplasmic regions, which are responsible for inducing and controlling specific cell wall synthesis. We, furthermore, received evidence that these developmental processes base on the nucleus. In this context, therefore, attention should be focussed on nucleus- dependent differentiation processes of the cytoplasm, especially of its marginal regions. In this context investigations on the development of the cysts appeared to be very promising, since it is easily possible to characterize the different developmental stages.
    Electron microscopic studies of cap rays, in which cytoplasmic compartition processes are already initiated, have shown a prominent increase of vesiculate bodies with special structural characteristics (see fig.3). In contrast to the roughly structured contents of the dictyosome vesicles their inclusions are nearly structureless. Up to now nothing is known about their chemical composition, and about their functions.
    When plasma compartition is completed, each compartment is delimited by a plasma membrane (see fig.3), and endoplasmic reticulum is aligned in parallel with it, thus indicating probable functional interrelationships. During these stages dictyosomes appear unusually structured, and intimately contact endoplasmic reticulum masses, which are unusual too. Only in few cases they possess the basic architecture that resembles to stalk or cap dictyosomes (fig.6, 7). Their terminal vesicles, however, are very small, and are comparable to those of low active dictyosomes of certain stalk regions of Acetabularia cells. Since dictyosomes are known to be involved in cell wall precursor polysaccharide synthesis for stalk or

cap wall formation in <u>Acetabularia</u>, their possible function in cyst wall formation is of special interest. But as it stands now, no indication was received for their participation in this process, which leads to a cell wall that is structurally and chemically different from the other cell walls of <u>Acetabularia</u>.

During these stages of cyst development, in which also the vesicular bodies show conspicuous alterations, a thin layer of cyst wall becomes appearant (fig.6, 7). By "influx" of new polysaccharides the cyst wall becomes progressive thickened, but remains relatively weak structured (see Werz 1968 a).

In some electron micrographs the possibility of a participation of certain regions of the plasma membrane in synthesizing cyst wall polysaccharide is indicated (see fig.6). The existence of cell wall polysaccharide synthesizing enzymes within the plasma membrane was demonstrated for yeast cells by Moor and Mühlethaler (1963). As is shown in figure 8, such enzyme complexes are part of the surface of the plasma membrane. But also in this case the question remains: how do these enzymes attain the membrane surface, and where are they synthesized?

Whereas all of these mechanisms are functioning in the nucleate system, they have never been observed to occur in an anucleate cytoplasm. As it was already demonstrated such cytoplasm is neither capable of forming plasma compartments, and therefore of forming the corresponding new plasma membranes, nor is it able to synthesize cyst wall, indicating the failure of the corresponding active enzymes. We, therefore, have to conclude that the differentiation of the special functional features of plasma membranes, responsible for the induction of cyst wall synthesis is governed by the nucleus. Moreover, it seems to be evident that the formation of plasma membranes and their supply with specific functions, i.e. enzymes, is not only a main basis for cell wall synthesis, but rather is a basic morphogenetic principle.

In cellulose cell wall formation the orientation of microfibrils probably is directed by microtubules (see Newcomb and Bonnett 1965). These cytoplasmic elements are sensitive to colchicine, that binds to their sub- unit proteins (see Borisy and Taylor 1967 a,b; Shelansky and Taylor 1967).

Colchicine- sensitivity is observed also in <u>Acetabularia</u>
cells at certain developmental stages, i.e. when a new
direction of growth has to be initiated. Stalk growth,
for instance, is not interferred by the alkaloid, while
it inhibits the formation of caps. It has been demonstrated that the interference of cap formation is not dependent on an inactivation of those mechanisms which determine species- specificity of the caps. It rather are certain non- species- specific "induction mechanisms"
which are inhibited by the alkaloid. If, therefore, cap
formation is already started, the cap's growth is normal
under the influence of the colchicine (see Werz 1969 a,b).
In the case of cyst development similar effects of colchicine were observed: when it is applied to the early
"two- dimensional" stages the further compartition of the
plasma is inhibited, and cell wall formation, therefore,
is suppressed. The continuation of cyst development,
however, is not affected, when the alkaloid is applied to
the "three- dimensional" plasma compartments (Werz 1969
a, b).
     Since colchicine is regarded to react specifically
with microtubular sub- unit proteins, not only the protein
-character of the inducing "agents" is obvious. It rather
points to the existence of such cytoplasmic elements in
those critical stages of development, which have been
found to be colchicine-sensitive. However, within the
cytoplasm of the critical developmental stages in question,
microtubules have not been detected. It is, therefore,
suggested that in the <u>Acetabularia</u> cell's morphogenesis
other structures are functioning, which nevertheless dispose of similar functions. As one possibility it may be
taken into consideration that non- aggregated microtubular
sub- units are present within the cytoplasmic regions in
question. Vague indications for the existence of "disor-
ganized" microtubules within the cytoplasm were received
from electron microscopic studies of zygote cells. They
have shown that microtubular constituents of the flagella are split into sub- units at the flagellar bases, and
are distributed over the cytoplasm before cell wall formation starts. However, as it stands now, neither evidence
was received that they exert specific functions in the
morphogenetic events, nor that they represent the col-
chicine- sensitive units of the cytoplasm, responsible

for inducing morphogenetic events.

Conclusions

The shape of a plant cell is not determined by the mode of the cell's wall growth. In <u>Acetabularia</u> it was demonstrated that it is the cytoplasm, which determines the cell's shape. It is, on the one hand, engaged in the fabrication of cell wall precursor polysaccharides, and on the other hand is determining the cell's shape by its ability to undergo morphogenesis. During these events, which are nucleus- dependent, a plasmatic "model" of a species- characteristic is developed. It disposes of specific functional properties in its peripheral cytoplasm. They induce and control the processing of cell wall precursor material into the diverse chemical and structural qualities of species- specific cell walls. It is proposed that the cytoplasmic "model" delimiting plasma membrane is basically involved in these events, thus playing an important role in the cell's morphogenesis.

References

1. J. Heslop- Harrison, <u>Science 161</u>, 230 (1968),
2. W. I. Nickerson, <u>Cellular Membranes in Development</u>, (M.Locke, ed.), Acad. Press New York and London. p. 281 (1964),
3. J. Hämmerling and K. Zetsche, <u>Umschau 66</u>, 489 (1966),
4. R.B. Bloch, <u>Handb. Pflanzenphysiol. XI/ 1</u>, Springer- Verlag Berlin- Heidelberg- New York, p. 146 (1965),
5. P.A. Roelofsen, Adv. Bot. Res. 2, 69 (1965),
6. J. Hämmerling, <u>Biol. Zbl. 59</u>, 158 (1939),
7. K. L. Schulze, <u>Arch. Protistenk. 92</u>, 179 (1939),
8. G. Werz, <u>Protoplasma 65</u>, 81 (1968 a),
9. G. Werz, <u>Protoplasma 65</u>, 349 (1968 b),
10. G. Werz, <u>Protoplasma 67</u>, 67 (1969 a),
11. G. Werz, <u>Inhibitors- Tools in Cell Research</u>, 20. Coll. Ges. Physiol. Chemie, Mosbach. Springer- Verlag Berlin- Heidelberg- New York (1969 b),

12. A. Gibor, Proc. Natl. Acad. Sci. (Wash.) 54,1527 (1965),
13. H. Moor and K. Mühlethaler, J. Cell Biol. 17,609 (1963),
14. E.H. Newcomb and H. T. Bonnett, J. Cell Biol. 27,575 (1965),
15. G.G. Borisy and E. W. Taylor, J. Cell Biol. 34, 525 (1967 a),
16. G.G. Borisy and E. W. Taylor, J. Cell Biol. 34, 535 (1967 b),
17. M.L. Shelansky and E. W. Taylor, J. Cell Biol. 34, 549 (1967).

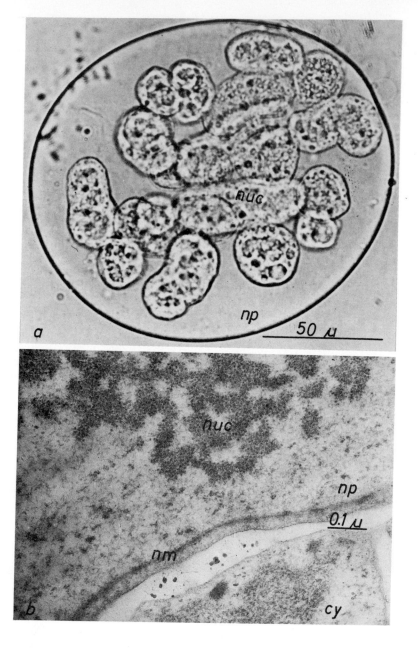

Figure 1. a) Living nucleus isolated from the rhizoid of Acetabularia mediterranea.

b) Electron micrograph of a nucleus of A. mediterranea fixed in glutaraldehyde-OsO$_4$, pH 7.2, and embedded in Maraglass, lead- stained. np = nucleoplasm, nuc = nucleoli, nm = nuclear envelope, cy = cytoplasm.

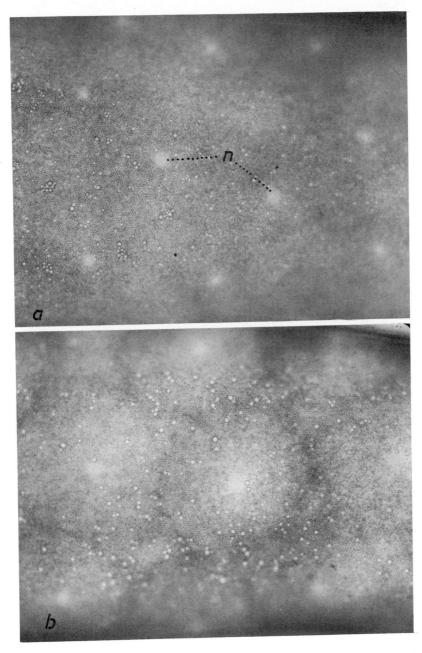

Figure 2. Successive stages of cytoplasmic morphogenesis during cyst development in the cap rays of A. (Polyphysa) cliftonii. a – d = plasma compartition processes, leading to the cytoplasmic cyst model (e), which is at least covered by cyst wall (f; cw). n = secondary nuclei. 143 x.

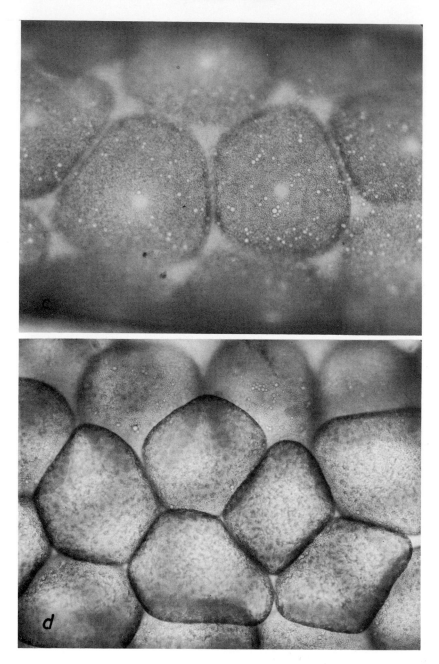

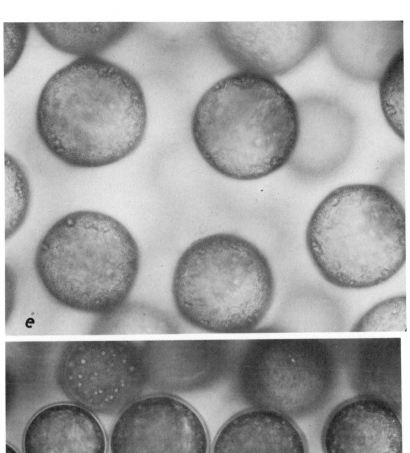

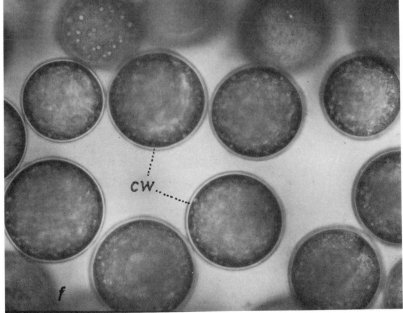

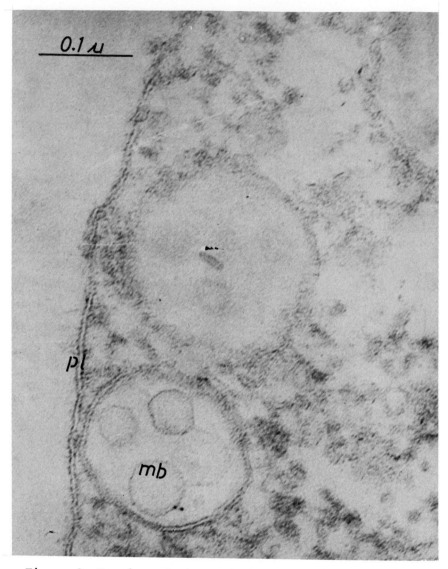

Figure 3. Portion of the periphery of the cytoplasmic cyst model, of A. (Polyphysa) cliftonii, showing the plasma membrane (pl), and vesicular bodies (mb). A cell wall is not yet present, but possibly starts to become synthesized at certain regions of the plasma membrane. Glutaraldehyde- OsO4 fixation, embedded in Epon- 812.

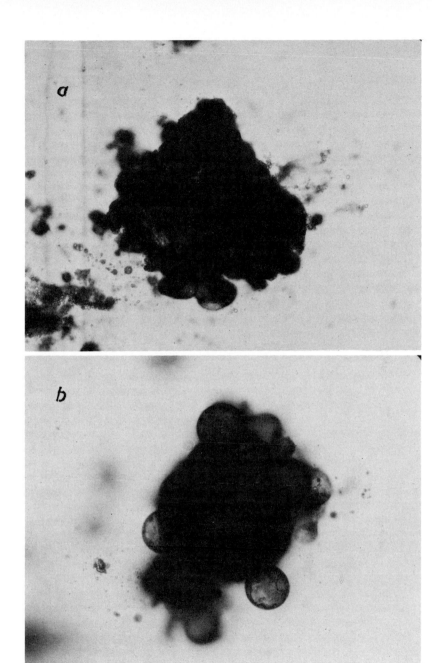

Figure 4. a - c . The morphogenetic behaviour of protoplasts from cap ray plasm of A. (Polyphysa) clif-tonii. They differentiate under in vitro conditions, and synthesize cyst wall (cw), that can be demonstrated by "staining" with chlorzink- iodine- reagent (d). 143 x.

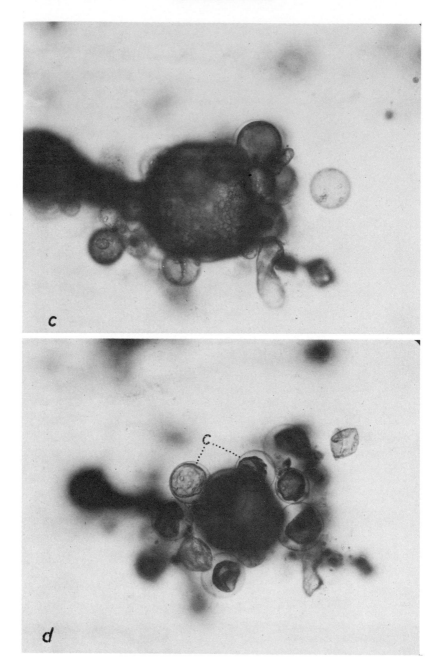

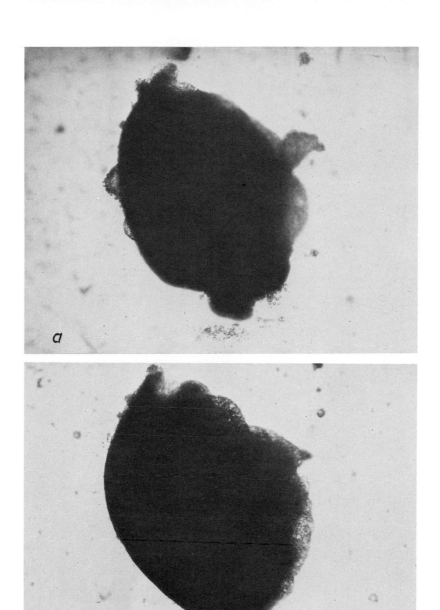

Figure 5. a – b. Cytoplast of cap ray plasm of A. (Polyphysa) cliftonii. Cytoplasts are in contrast to the protoplasts never capable of differentiating "cysts" and of
synthesizing cell wall. They only alter their shape by
movements of the cytoplasm. 153 x.

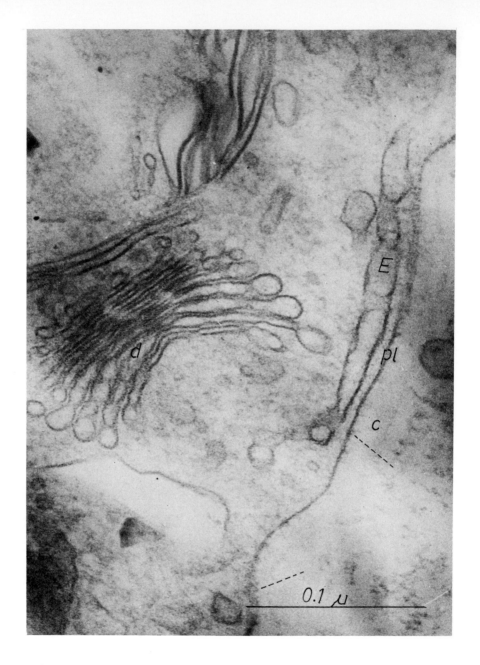

Figure 6. A. (Polyphysa) cliftonii. A small layer of cyst wall (c) is deposited upon the plasma membrane (pl). E = endoplasmic reticulum, d = dictyosome, ------ = possible regions of cell wall microfibril synthesis. $KMnO_4$- fixed; embedded in Epon-812.

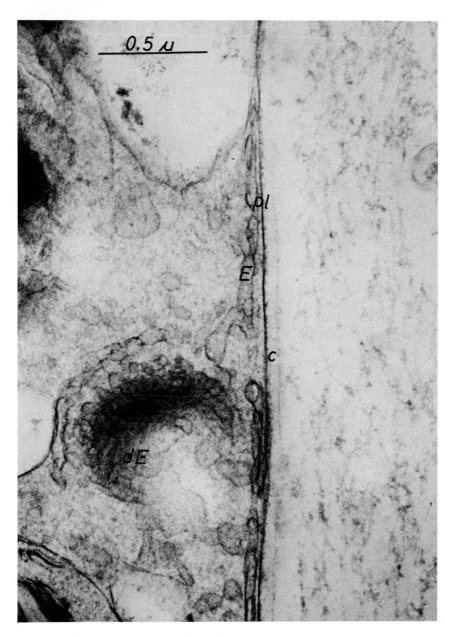

Figure 7. A. (Polyphysa) cliftonii. A layer of cyst wall
is formed upon the plasma membrane (pl). c = cyst wall,
E = endoplasmic reticulum, partially connected with endoplasmic reticulum masses associated with dictyosomes (dE).
KMnO$_4$- fixation, embedded in Epon- 812.

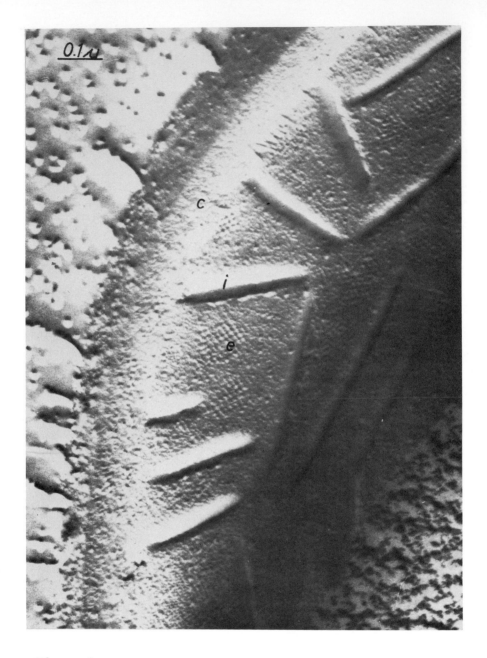

Figure 8. Freeze- etching preparation of the surface of the plasma membrane of yeast. Besides distinct invaginations (i), enzyme complexes (e) can be observed. They were shown to partake in the synthesis of cell wall polysaccharides by Moor and Mühlethaler (1963). c = cell wall. Original Dr. Kellner.

ULTRASTRUCTURE OF ACETABULARIA MEDITERRANEA IN THE COURSE OF FORMATION OF THE SECONDARY NUCLEI

Monique Boloukhère

Laboratory of Animal Morphology, Free University of Brussels, Brussels, Belgium.

Abstract

The ultrastructure of the rhizoïds of Acetabularia mediterranea has been studied on algae which have performed the outgrowth of the cap.

Electron micrographs of algae whose primary nucleus seems unchanged, suggest that young chloroplasts are being formed in the perinuclear cytoplasm. They seem to arise by a constriction of old chloroplasts filled with storage granules. Some of the newly formed chloroplasts also appear to multiply. They give rise to proplastid-like organelles and afterwoods degenerate. The others unchanged young chloroplasts migrate with the secondary nuclei.

The mitochondria of the perinuclear area show processes which might reflect a multiplication of these organelles. The increase in cytoplasmic basophilia is due to the presence of nuclear fragments containing part of the fragmented nucleolus. The loss of density of the nucleolus in the primary nucleus is related to the disappearance of a fibrillar component, to the vacuolization of the central zone and to the emission of spherules. It leads to the formation of a granular ring structure.

No mitotic figures were observed. Moreover, we noted in the nucleoplasm groups of irregular nodosities clustered along broad-thread like structures. Each nodosity was found to be composed of coiled fibers.

Symbols: DNA = desoxyribonucleic acid; RNA = ribonucleic acid.

The secondary nuclei (about 5 μ) formed in the rhizoïds, lack the buds as well as the cytoplasmic border. They contain a single nucleolus and chromatin located in the nucleoplasm.

Examination of the cytoplasm shows the presence of bundles of microtubules : their role is unknown.

The possible signification of these observations is discussed in terms of nucleocytoplasmic relationships, with respect to the life cycle of Acetabularia mediterranĕa.

Introduction

As Schultze (26) has shown with the optical microscope, the primary nucleus situated in the rhizoïds is pulverized into a series of secondary nuclei, when the cap of the alga has reached a certain size. The only external visible sign of this activity is the lightening of the color of the siphon which becomes pale green.
Micrographs are presented to show the appearance of the cytoplasm of the rhizoïds from algae at this stage. The changes undergone by the primary nucleus are reported. Secondary nuclei could be observed. Their ultrastructure and that of the surrounding cytoplasm, is described.

Material and methods

Algae were chosen when cap formation was finished and when the cytoplasm of the siphon was beginning to become clear. All operations were completed at room temperature. The cells were fixed with 6% glutaraldehyde buffered with 0,1 M phosphate (pH = 7,4) for 24 hours. After a period of fixation of 10 minutes to half an hour, the cells are cut into two fragments, in order to facilitate the fixation and, later on, the embedding. The fragments were washed three times over a hour period, in 0,1 M phosphate buffer and then postfixed with 1 % osmium tetroxyde in phosphate buffer for 1 hour. The osmium tetroxyde is eliminated by washing the material three times for a period of fifteen minutes in 0,1 M phosphate buffer. The fragments of the algae are dehydrated in a graded series of alcohols, embedded in epon and sectioned with glass knives. The specimen were cut transversally to the axis of the si-

146

phon. The block was then retrimmed under the binocular leaving a square containing little else but the nucleus. All sections were doubly stained at room temperature, with aqueous uranyl acetate (4 %) for 17 to 20 hours and lead citrate for 20 minutes. Micrographs were taken on an AEI type EM6B microscope.

Results

Chloroplasts

In the rhizoïds of an alga whose vegetative nucleus is not yet fragmented (Figure 1), some sections of chloroplasts show a translucent stroma and a lamellar system organized into well differentiated pseudogranar and interpseudogranar regions. Nevertheless, most of them show, in addition to the lamellar system, one (Figure 1), sometimes several carbohydrate storage granules. It is appearent from the sections that there are at least two types of chloroplasts. When the grains within the chloroplasts are large, they are stacked in big spheroïd chloroplasts (Figure 1), as generally observed in the rhizoïds (32). Otherwise these grains are lined up in elongated chloroplasts, resembling those of the basal portion of the siphon (Figure 2). In this second type of chloroplasts, one sometimes observes a fibrillar region which resembles the DNA containing regions described by Werz (35) and Puiseux-Dao et al. (23, 24). In favorable cases the section shows that the chloroplast is putting forth a bud in the neighbouring region (Figure 3). There are good indications of a contact between the bud and the DNA containing region (Figure 3). In all cases, these buds show a granular stroma, a major lamellar system and numerous osmiophilic globules, but no storage granule (Figure 4). They appear to be of variable size. The observation of constriction figures (Figure 5) suggests the separation of the lamellar bud from the rest of the chloroplast. This hypothesis seems to be confirmed by the appearance in the cytoplasm of new chloroplasts, with a structure identical to that of the lamellar buds (Figure 6). The only difference lies in the hypertrophy of the lamellar system which exists in the new chloroplasts. In the budding chloroplasts, bundles of lamellae occur which differ slightly

147

in appearance from those usually observed. They will be referred to as "rods" (Figure 5, 7). They have a diameter of 130 to 200 nm and may attain a lenght of several μ. They sometimes form rows of an almost crystalline inclusion. At high magnification, they appear to be made of dense granules about 170 nm in diameter, some of which sometimes lie free in the stroma (5). Some of the newly formed chloroplasts are probably compressed in their median region into a bell shape, since some of them probably cut transversally to the bell axis (Figure 7) seem to be ring shaped, while others, probably cut parallel to the bell axis appear to be U shaped (Figure 8). During the fragmentation of the primary nucleus, the number of cup-shaped chloroplasts increases. The hyaloplasm enclosed within the bell or cup of the chloroplast contains many more ribosomes than the surrounding cytoplasm ; these ribosomes are often arranged in clusters. Occasionally, such cup-shaped chloroplasts appear to put forth structures which look like proplastids, on the basis of both of their own dimensions (about 1 μ) and those of the osmiophilic globules (30-130 nm), which they enclose (Figure 8). The proplastid-like structures form on contact with the lamellae of the chloroplasts. They enclose the osmiophilic globules of the chloroplasts. They bud towards the exterior of the chloroplast (Figure 9), where they are ultimately liberated (Figure 9). During this process, the stroma of the cup-shaped chloroplasts becomes finely fibrillar. These chloroplasts remain in the rhizoïds where they degenerate, while the other unmodified chloroplasts migrate with the secondary nuclei (Figure 17).

Mitochondria

When the primary nucleus remains unchanged the cytoplasm contains ribosomes and typical mitochondria recognizable by their cristae and their dense granules (Figure 1). In the neighbourhood of a nuclear fragment, numerous mitochondria appear, which are very similar to those usually found in the rhizoïds (Figure 10). Most of them are clustered in strings of beads. Some larger mitochondria appear also at this stage. These latter show curved cristae which are particularly long (Figure 11). They are connected or just in contact with buds which strongly recall the newly formed mitochondria by their size and appearance.

Microtubules

In the cytoplasm surrounding the fragmenting nucleus, bundles of microtubules can be seen, orientated parallel to the axis of the siphon. They are never encountered in the neighbourhood of an organelle. Later on, during the migration of the secondary nuclei, bundles of microtubules appear which in this case, run perpendicular to the axis of the siphon (Figure 17). Profiles of these are sometimes seen to be packed together adjacent to the secondary nuclei (Figure 17).

Inclusions

At this stage, the rhizoïds show numerous osmiophilic granules about 1 μ in diameter identified by Werz (34) as polyphosphate granules (Figure 1). It has been shown, that processes of phosphorylation (28) are involved in the synthesis of different types of polyphosphates, according to the state of polymerisation (30).

Primary nucleus

The primary nucleus possesses a double nuclear membrane with wavy contours. This membrane is surrounded by a cytoplasmic border (7,32). From this border emerge buds which are called "nuclear emissions" (7, 32, 33, 34). They contain ribosomes , as previously illustrated (32). In addition, they sometimes show spherical heterogenous bodies, which appear to be composed of several fibrillar regions packed together with a few granules. However, at this stage, in the perinuclear cytoplasm, the most prominent fact is the abundance of buds which look like replicae of the nuclear membrane. The nucleus often forms lobules, which separate from the rest of the nucleus. When these lobules break away from the nucleus, they may carry with them fragments of the nucleolus. In some sections the nucleolus may still resemble that of a full grown alga (Figure 12) ; it has a central region consisting of fibrils of 50 to 100 nm in diameter and a cortical region mainly composed of granules of about 200 nm. The central region is organized into a hollow cylinder from which centripetal structures expand. Whether or not the granules of the cortical zone do in fact

represent kinks of the fibrils cannot be decided from our
micrographs. In the region of interpenetration small round
vacuoles exist. The central region contains a single irregular vacuole, which is invaded by fibrillar structures.
However, serial sections have been made in about ten nuclei. They show the degenerative changes which are related
to the loss of density of the nucleolus (Figure 13). They
indicate the progressive disappearance of the fibrillar
zone of the nucleolus. The fibrillar structures of the
nucleolus seem to condense and to disappear first. Figure
13 shows a nucleolus with a greatly reduced fibrillar zone.
The centripetal structures have now disappeared from the
central vacuole. Part of this fibrillar material seems to
be scattered in the form of spherules. Part of the granular material also seems to be scattered in the form of
spherules. Both types of spherules are observed in the
nucleolus and in the nucleoplasm (Figure 13). When they
are located in the neighbourhood of the nuclear membrane,
serial sections suggest that contact occurs not only between the two types of spherules, but also between them
and two new types of spherules. The latter are characterized by a coarser fibred texture (Figure 14). On many
micrographs (Figure 15) the fibrillar zone has totally
disappeared. Vacuoles appear in the central zone. At their
level, the material is more dispersed. These vacuoles se-
condarily acquire more precise contours through the appearance, on their surface, of granules similar to those
of the nucleolar cortical zone. These granules might very
well originate in the cortical zone of the nucleolus.
Indeed during the invasion of the central zone by clusters
of granules, condensation of the reticulo-granular zone
occurs. These processes lead to the formation of ring
structures, which contain exclusively the granular component of the nucleolus. Mitotic figures are absent from the
nucleoplasm at this stage. Instead, broad thread-like
structures appear, between 0,2 and 0,3 μ in diameter and
of variable length. These structures are composed of irregular nodosities, which seem to be formed by involuted
fibrils (Figure 16).

Secondary nuclei and surrounding cytoplasm

The secondary nuclei are limited by a double nuclear membrane, which lacks the border and the cytoplasmic buds which characterize the primary nucleus (Figures 17, 18). They posses a nucleolus which has a dense reticulated region and a central region less dense to electrons. The nucleolus is different from that of the primary nucleus, since it is composed of two fibrillar constituents. In the nucleoplasm clumps of chromatin are generally visible (Figure 18). They consist of fibers about 100 nm, in diameter, which seem to form loose spirals. Under phase contrast, light microscope, one can observe in this type of nucleus short-paired segments suggesting a prophase state. However, other secondary nuclei are characterized by the occurence of condensed perinucleolar chromatin (Figure 17). A granular mass is nearly always associated with the nucleus (Figure 18). The structure and appearance of this mass recall the nuclear emissions which are present in the cytoplasm surrounding the primary nucleus. As already indicated, the surrounding cytoplasm contains new young chloroplasts (Figure 17). Dictyosomes and ribosomes (Figure 18) are also present. The latter are arranged in clusters. When they are attached to membranes, they confer upon the latter the aspect of a endoplasmic reticulum. In addition, microtubules are aggregated into bundles, orientated here perpendicular to the axis of the siphon (Figure 17).

Discussion

When the primary nucleus remains unchanged, electron micrographs show the formation of lamellar buds and their growth and separation from the rest of the chloroplasts. One can therefore postulate the formation of young chloroplasts by the constriction of old chloroplasts filled with storage granules. In the latter, during the process of budding, the rods and quasi-crystalline arrangements of granules recall the observations of Bartels and Weier (2) on the proplastids of Triticum vulgare. According to these authors, these inclusions are due to the synthesis of membranes on ribosomes which are attached to them. In Acetabularia, they could also be related to the development of the membrane system. This would explain the origin of the hypertrophied membrane system described in the new young chlororoplast.

151

Some of the new chloroplasts acquire a cup-shaped
form. This cup-shaped form, also called the umbo-form,
exists in others plasts. Woodcock and Bell (36) observed
it in Ranunculacea (Myosorus) at the time of the formation
of the female gametophyte. They interpreted it as a sign
of very rapid reproduction of the organelles. In Acetabularia this umbo-form of the young chloroplasts might also
accompany their reproduction. The budding of structures
resembling proplastids strengthens this hypothesis. There
thus seems to be an active multiplication of the chloroplasts of Acetabularia. It apparently occurs in two successive phases, the first consisting in the constriction of
old chloroplasts filled with storage granules and the second in the budding of new chloroplasts. The mitochondria
seem to be affected by the fragmentation of the primary
nucleus. They exhibit figures which recall the different
stages of growth and mitochondrial multiplication described by Manton (19) in Anthoceros and by Tandler and al (29)
in mouse hepathic cells. Thus the micrographs which we have
shown suggest that cytoplasmic rejuvenation occurs by the
active multiplication of chloroplasts and mitochondria.
Examination of the cytoplasm has shown the presence of
bundles of microtubules. In other material, different
authors have assigned to them a role in plant membrane synthesis (37, 14), in ion transport (21), in protoplasmic
streamings (17) or even in mitosis (15, 25). In Acetabularia, it is impossible to attribute any precise role to
these structures as yet. The only well established fact is
that they appear just at the time when cellular movement
occurs, i.e. migration and mitoses of the secondary nuclei.
The numerous polyphosphate granules encountered in the cytoplasm are thought to reflect the importance of processes
of oxydative phosphorylation at this stage (28). Observations made by Schultze (26) and Vanderhaeghe (31) under the
light microscope, have shown that the desintegration of the
primary nucleus parallels an increase of basophilia in the
cytoplasm. Ultrastructural studies suggest that this phenomenon is probably due to the pinching off of lobules, which
separate from the nucleus carrying with them part of the
nucleolus. The loss of density of the nucleolus, noted by
the same author seems to be related to the disappearance of
the fibrillar component and to a vacuolization of the central zone. It leads to the formation of a granular ring

structure probably similar to the "Restkörper" described
by Schultze. Like this author, we have never observed
mitotic figures at this stage. The beginning of the invo-
lution of the fibrils in the nucleoplasm could maybe indicate the onset of the individualization of the chromosomes. In fact their appearance coïncides with that of the
light pink Feulgen staining of the nucleoplasm noted by
Puiseux-Dao (22). Early light—microscopic observations
(31) have revealed the existence of two types of secondary
nuclei. Our micrographs are consistent with this view.
In the first type, the presence of the nucleolus and the
presence of twin strands suggest a true prophase. In the
second type, the condensed perinucleolar chromatin may
correspond to the onset of the individualization of the
chromosomes. The nucleus would thus perhaps be in early
prophase.

The micrographs concerning the desintegration of the
nucleolus recall those of actinomycin treated algae. They
suggest a drop in activity of the nucleus under the influence of a natural repressor of RNA synthesis. The differenciation of organelles like chloroplasts and mitochondria proceeds simultaneously. These findings are consistent with the view that these organelles show a high degree of autonomy towards the nucleus. As pointed out by
autoradiographic (3), chemical (6, 12, 13, 16) and by
cytochemical (1, 10, 11, 27) experiments, this autonomy is
linked to the presence of replicating DNA in these organelles. Recent preliminary unpublished data (18) indicate
unusual amounts of cytoplasmic DNA at this stage. Such
findings could be accounted for by the differenciation of
the new cytoplasmic organelles. A similar reconstitution
of the cytoplasm has been observed by various authors
(9, 20, 36) at the time of formation of the gametes such
as for example, the egg cell of a fern (Pteridium), the
gametophyte of a moss (Sphaerocarpus) or the gametophyte
of a primitive angiosperm (Myosorus). It has been interpreted by these authors as a preparation of the cytoplasm
for the haploïd phase of the gametophyte. It could signify,
that at the end of the vegetative life of Acetabularia, a
new generation of chloroplasts and mitochondria arises,
destinated for the cytoplasm of the gametes in the cysts.

References

1. E. Baltus and J. Brachet, Biochim. Biophy. Acta 61, 157, 1962.
2. P. G. Bartels and T. E. Weier, J.Cel. Biol. 33 243, 1967.
3. J. Brachet, Exp. Cell Res. suppl. 6, 73, 1959.
4. M. Bol64khère, J. Microscopie 4, 363, 1965.
5. M. Bol64khère, sous presse 1969.
6. C. J. Chapman N. A. Nugent and R. W. Schreiber, Plant. Physiol. 41, 589, 1966.
7. J.C.W. Crawley, Exp. Cell Res. 32, 368, 1963.
8. F. de Vitry, Bull. Soc. Chim. Biol. 47, 1325, 1965.
9. Diers, Organisation der Zelle. Springer-Verlag Berlin, 227, 1966.
10. A. Gibor and M. Izawa, Proc.Nat.Acad. Sci. U.S. 50, 1164, 1963.
11. A. Gibor, Biochemistry of Chloroplasts, Goodwin II,321 1967.
12. V. Heilporn and J. Brachet, Biochim. Biophys. Acta, 119, 429, 1966.
13. B. Green V. Heilporn S. Limbosch M. Bol64khère and J. Brachet, Proc. Nat. Acad. Sci. U.S. 58, 1351, 1967.
14. P. K. Hepler and E.H. Newcomb, J. Cell Biol. 20, 529, 1964.
15. P. K. Hepler and W. T. Jackson, J. Cell Biol. 38, 437, 1968.
16. M. Janowski, Biochim. Biophys. Acta, 103, 399, 1965.
17. M. C. Ledbetter and K. R. Porter, J. Cell Biol. 29, 239, 1963.
18. S. Limbosch and V. Heilporn, unpublished results, 1969.
19. I. Manton, J. Exp. Bot. 12, 421, 1961.
20. Ph D. Mühlethaler and P. R. Bell, J. Cell Biol. 20, 235, 1968.
21. J. Pochon-Masson, Année Biol. IV, (7-8) 1967.
22. S. Puiseux-Dao, Thèse, série A, n° 3879, 1962.
23. S. Puiseux-Dao and D. Hoursiangou-Neubrun, 6th Inter. Con. Electr. Microsc. Kyoto, 2, 331, 1966.

24. S. Puiseux-Dao, D. Gibello and D. Hoursiangou-Neubrun, C.R. Acad. Sci. Paris, 265, 406, 1967.
25. L. E. Roth, Primitive motile systems in Cell Biology 527 (R.D. Allen N. Kamiya, Eds Ac.Pr. N. Y. 647, pp). 1964.
26. K. Schultze, Arch. Protist. 92, 179, 1939.
27. D. Shephard, Exp. Cell Res. 37, 93, 1965.
28. H. Stich, Z. Naturforsch. 10b, 281, 1955.
29. B. Tandler, R.A. Erlandson, A. L. Smith and E.L. Wynder, J. Cell Biol. 41, 477, 1969.
30. E. Thilo, H. Grunze, J. Hämmerling and G. Werz, Z. Naturforsch. 11b, 266, 1956.
31. F. Vanderhaeghe, Thèse. non publiée. 1957.
32. P. Van Gansen et M. Boloukhère, J. Microscopie 4 347, 1965.
33. G. Werz, Z.Naturforsch. 16b, 126, 1961.
34. G. Werz, Planta 62, 255, 1964.
35. G. Werz, Planta 68, 256, 1966.
36. C. L. F. Woodcock and P.R. Bell. J. Ultr. Res. 22, 546, 1968.
37. F.B.P. Wooding and D.H. Northcote. J. Cell Biol. 23, 327, 1964.

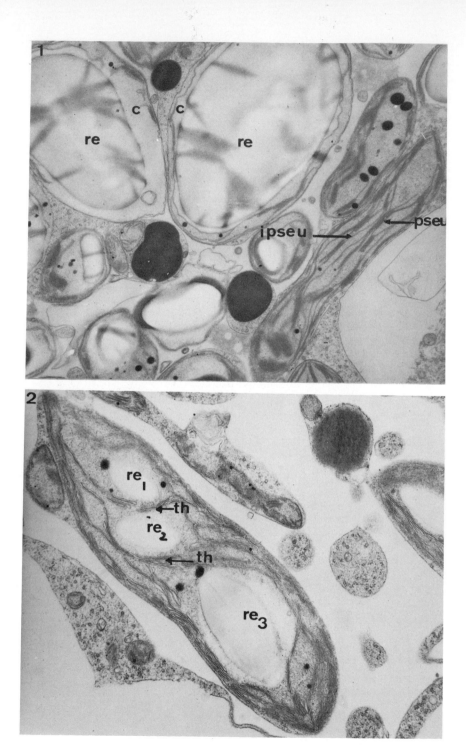

Figures 1-7.Views of the cytoplasm situated in the rhizoïds of an alga whose vegetative nucleus is not yet
fragmented.

Figure 1.
Some sections of chloroplasts show the lamellar system
which is organized into well differenciated pseudogranar
(pseu) and inter-pseudogranar (ipseu) regions. Other sections of chloroplasts show the carbohydrate storage granule (re) which here appears in a spheroïd chloroplast
(c). x 17.000

Figure 2.
A section of an elongated chloroplast showing carbohydrate storage granules (re_1, re_2, re_3) lined up and separated from each other by thylacoïds (th). x 17.000

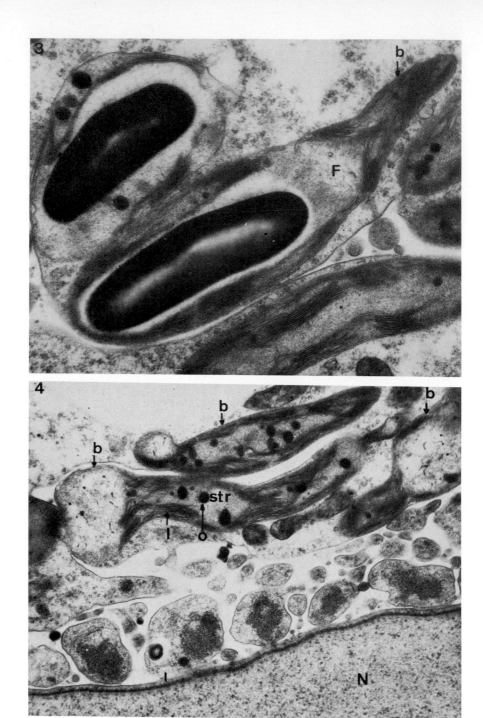

Figure 3.
A section of an elongated chloroplast showing clearly
the contact between the bud (b) and the fibrillar region
(F) resembling a DNA region. x 25.000

Figure 4.
The buds contain a granular stroma (str), osmiophilic
globules (o) and an important lamellar system (l). To the
figure, the clearly visible nucleus (N) enables us to lo-
cate the buds (b) in the perinuclear cytoplasm. x 15.000

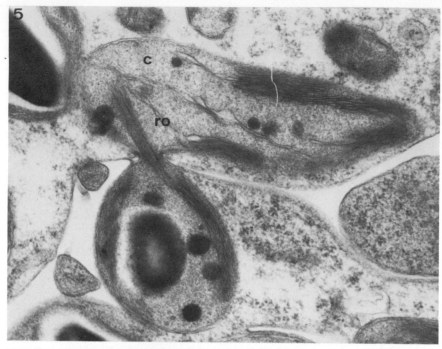

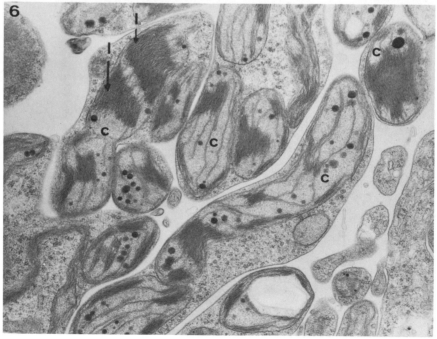

Figure 5.
A section showing a constriction figure (c) within a budding chloroplast. Bundles of lamellae occur, which differ
slightly in appearance from those usually observed.
They are referred to as " rods " (ro). x 30.000

Figure 6.
New chloroplasts (c) appear in the cytoplasm. The size
and morphology of these chloroplasts are similar to
those of the chloroplastic buds, except that the former
contain an hypertrophied lamellar system (1). x 15.000

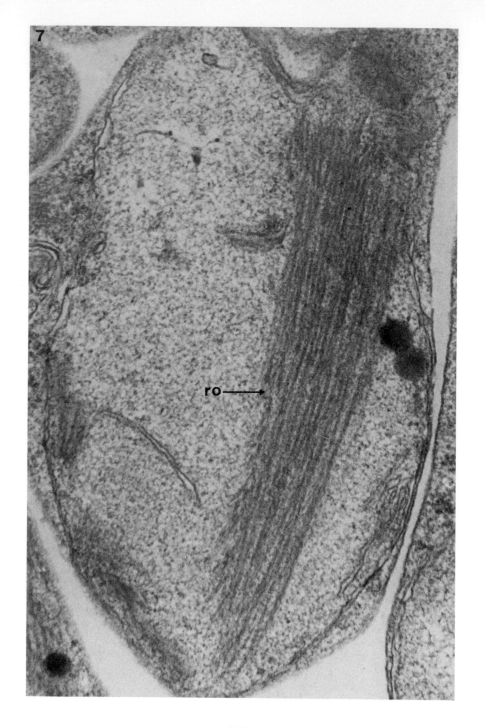

Figure 7.
A section of a budding chloroplast showing rods (ro) ar-
rayed in parallel rows. x 70.000

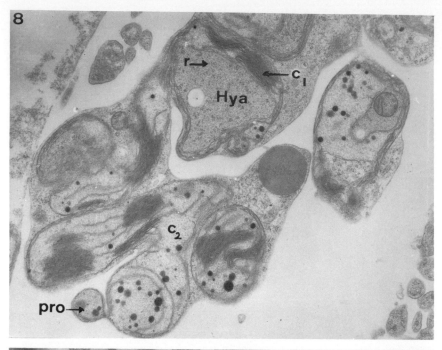

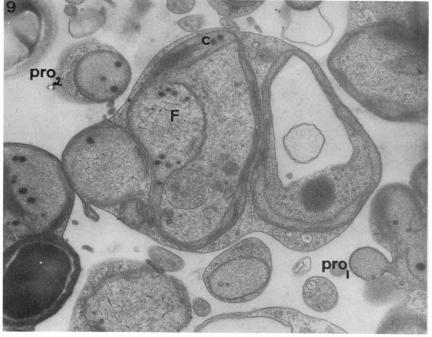

<u>Figures 8-11</u>. Views of the cytoplasm situated in the rhizoids of an alga whose vegetative nucleus is undergoing fragmentation.

<u>Figure 8</u>.
Newly formed chloroplasts which are probably cut transversally to the bell axis, seem to be ring shaped (c_1). Other newly formed chloroplasts which are probably cut parallel to the bell axis appear to be U shaped (c_2). The hyaloplasm (Hya) enclosed within the cup of the chloroplast contains clusters of ribosomes (r). Occasionally, such cup-shaped chloroplasts appear to put forth structures which look like proplastids (pro). x 15.000

<u>Figure 9</u>.
The section shows a cup-shaped chloroplast (c) with a fibrillar region (R) resembling the DNA region. A proplastid like structure is budding towards the exterior of the chloroplast (pro_1) while an other lies free in the cytoplasm (pro_2). x 15.000

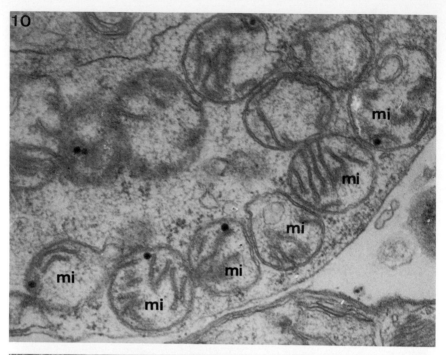

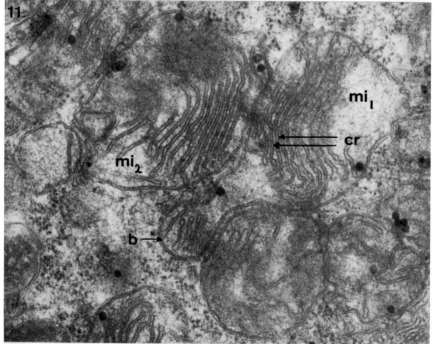

166

Figure 10.
New mitochondria (mi) appear clustered in strings of
beads in the neighbourhood of a nuclear fragment. x
40.000

Figure 11.
Some larger mitochondria (mi) are also present. They
have curved cristae (cr) which are particularly long.
One of them (mi$_1$) is forming a bud (b) resembling a
mitochondria of a normal size. An other one (mi$_2$) seems
in contact with a newly formed mitochondria. x 40.000

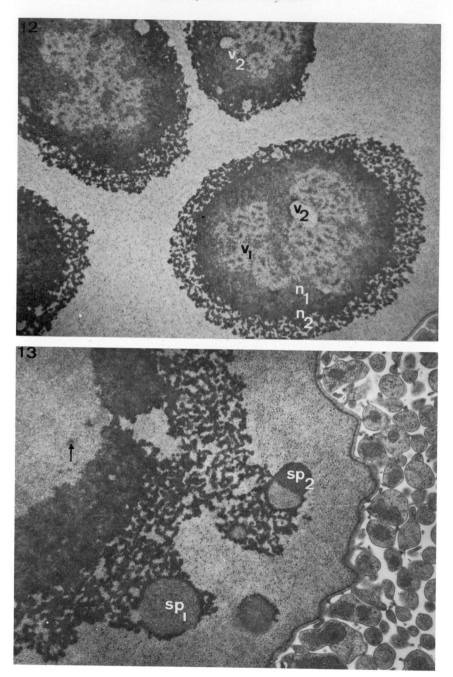

Figures 12-16. Transformation of the primary nucleus.

Figure 12.
The nucleolus shows a central region consisting of fi-
brils (n_1) and a cortical zone composed of granules (n_2).
The central zone contains a single irregular vacuole (v_1).
In the region of interpenetration small round vacuoles
(v_2) exist. x 17.000

Figure 13.
During the desintegration of the nucleolus, the fibrillar
centripetal structures first seem to disappear (see arrow). Both fibrillar (sp_1) and granular (sp_2) spherules
are scattered in the nucleoplasm. x 17.000

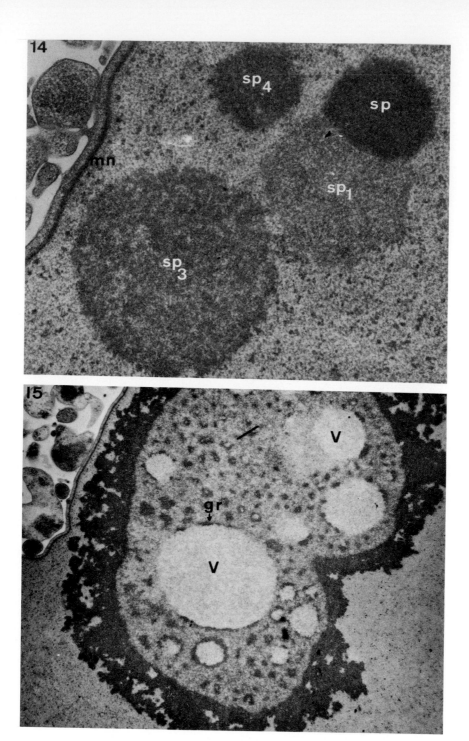

Figure 14.
When the spherules (sp_1 and sp_2) are located near the nuclear membrane (mn) they are in contact with two new types of spherules characterized by a coarser fibred texture (sp_3 and sp_4). x 30.000

Figure 15.
On this section the fibrillar material of the nucleolus has totally disappeared. Vacuoles (V) appear in the central zone. They acquire precise contours through the appearance on their surface of granules (gr) similar to those of the nucleolar cortical zone. x 17.000

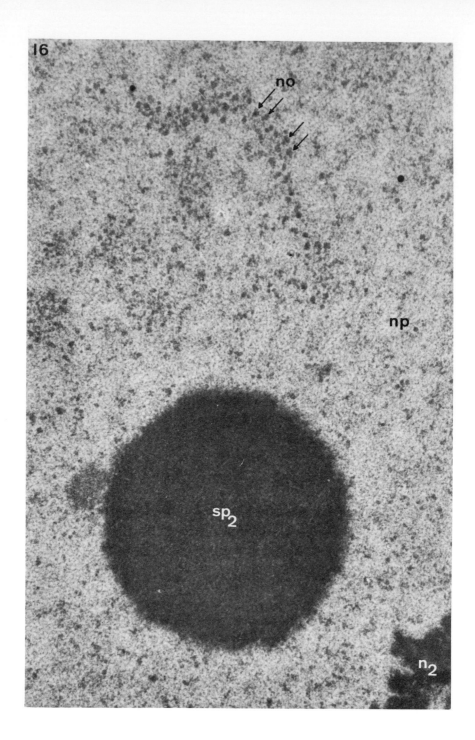

Figure 16.
A part of the nucleolus (n_2) is visible as well as a granular spherule (sp_2). The nucleoplasm (np) presents broad thread-like structures (see arrow) composed of irregular clustered nodosities (np). x 30.000

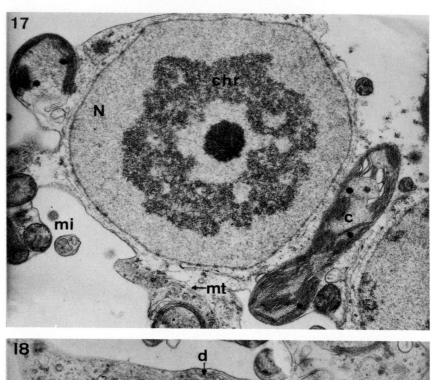

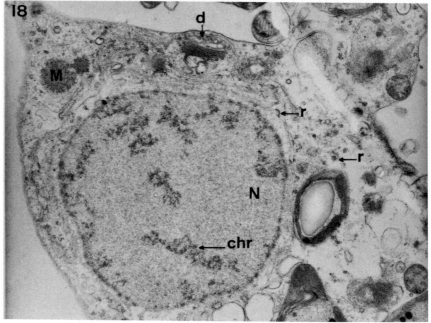

Figures 17-18. General views of the secondary nuclei formed in the rhizoïds and of the cytoplasm surrounding them.

Figure 17.
In this type of secondary nucleus (N), the chromatin fibers (chr) are condensed into a ring around the nucleolus
(n) from which only the dense reticulate zone is visible.
The perinuclear cytoplasm contains a new young mitochondrion (mi). x 15.000

Figure 18.
In this type of secondary nucleus (N), the slightly involuted chromatin fibers (chr) are aggregated in clumps.
A granular mass (M) is nearly always associated with the
nucleus. The perinuclear cytoplasm shows dictyosomes (d)
and ribosomes (r). x 15.000

EFFECT OF RED AND BLUE LIGHT ON MORPHOGENESIS AND METABOLISM OF <u>ACETABULARIA MEDITERRANEA</u>

Heins Clauss

Pflanzenphysiologisches Institut der Freien
Universität Berlin,
Berlin, Germany.

Abstract

A survey is given of the effect of red and blue light on morphogenesis, photosynthesis and metabolism of <u>Acetabularia mediterranea</u>. Growth ceases in red light almost completely after 2 - 3 weeks. This effect is mainly due to a decrease in the rate of photosynthesis. The reduction of the rate of photosynthesis is the result of changes, very probably, within the chloroplast, since Hill activity of chloroplast isolated from cells in red light also decreases with time. These different processes are reversible in blue light. Data are presented on the incorporation of ^{14}C during the reinduction of photosynthesis in blue light, following pretreatment with red light and on the distribution of ^{14}C on the different fractions.

Introduction

The morphogenesis of <u>Acetabularia</u> is strongly affected by light intensity. As shown by Beth [1] and later on by Terborgh and Thimann [2] high light intensity favours especially cap formation, while stalk growth is promoted by lower intensity. In order to interpret his results Beth assumes that perhaps different pigment systems might be involved and Mohr [3] attributes the high intensity reaction, i.e. cap formation to the blue region of the spectrum and the low energy reaction, i.e. growth of the stalk, to red light. Results published by Richter [4] seem

177

to confirm this supposition. He found, preferably with
Acetabularia crenulata, cap formation in blue light, in
red light, however, only in the order of 10% after 4
months.

Growth and photosynthesis in red and blue light

A reexamination on the effect of blue and red light
on the growth of Acetabularia yields a modified picture.
It was shown by Clauss (5) for Acetabularia mediterranea
and later on by Terborgh (6) for Acetabularia crenulata
that in red light ($\sim$ 600 - 700 nm) the growth rate decreases and ceases almost completely after about 2 - 3 weeks.
On the other hand, in blue light (350 - 500 nm) the cells
grow "normally" and form caps as they do in white light
(Fig. 1).

Obviously, red light does not inhibit cap formation
directly, since Acetabularia mediterranea cells in the
stage "just before cap formation" do form caps in red light,
within a short period following transfer to red light (5).
Furthermore, cells in red light may form caps in the order
of 1 per cent or less, provided they grow under these conditions, but with a restricted rate. These results support
the assumption that the failure of cap formation is mainly
the result of a general reduction of growth processes.

The reduction of growth in red light is accompanied
by a gradual drop of the rate of photosynthesis. In blue
light, as one may expect, for a growing cell, the O_2-evo-
lution per cell is slightly increasing (Fig. 2).
The effect of red light on photosynthesis is reversible
(7, 8). A transfer from continuous red light to continuous
blue light gives rise to an increase in the rate of photosynthesis within about 3 days up to the level in blue
light (Fig. 2). At the same time cells start to grow again
and if they have the appropriate stalk length they form
caps within $\sim$ 48 hours (4, 5). To reinduce growth and photosynthesis after red light treatment continuous blue light
may be substituted by giving short breaks of blue light in
addition to continuous red light (5, 6, 8).

Since in Acetabularia there is a close connection
between photosynthesis and growth, each influence on photosynthesis will finally effect growth processes. For this
reason the effect of red and blue light, respectively, on

178

cell growth is not surprising.

At present it is not known, whether in Acetabularia mediterranea there is a specific influence of blue light on growth and morphogenesis in addition to the indirect one via photosynthesis. To demonstrate such a specific effect in Acetabularia mediterranea is pretty difficult, but some results of similar experiments with another species, Acetabularia calyculus, point to this possibility (7).

Effect of red and blue light on Hill activity

Since changes in the rate of photosynthesis are involved in this light effect, it seems very likely that these are caused by an alteration of the photosynthetic machinery within the chloroplast. In order to get an idea whether this assumption is correct, the Hill activity of chloroplasts, isolated from cells grown in red and blue light, respectively, was determined. In accordance with the decrease in the rate of photosynthesis, there is a decrease in Hill activity (reduction of trichlorophenol indophenol, reference figure: chlorophyll). After 2 weeks in red light Hill activity is only about 1/3 to 1/4 of the value of chloroplasts isolated from cells grown under blue light conditions. Also in this case, returning the cells from red to blue light results in an increase of Hill activity within about 3 days up to the level of chloroplasts isolated from cells grown in blue light. It is concluded that under red light conditions there are some changes within the chloroplasts. Apparently, after red light treatment the chloroplasts have a reduced capacity to form "reduction equivalents" compared with cells grown in blue light. This is probably the main reason for the lower photosynthetic activity in red light. It is still unknown, whether red light acts directly on the chloroplasts or indirectly via the cytoplasm.

Influence of light quality on the photosynthetic ^{14}C-fixation

In order to get some information about the biochemical processes, accompanying these light effects, some experiments on ^{14}C-incorporation were performed. Cells were grown for various times in continuous red and blue light of an intensity of about 4000 erg cm^{-2}sec^{-1} and were allowed to photosynthate for 120 min in the presence of ^{14}C as NaHCO$_3$ in white light under conditions of light saturation (ca. 800 ftc). It will be shown later on, that this irradation for 2 hours with white light, will not enhance ^{14}C-incorporation. After 2 h of photosynthesis cells were fractionated into the following fractions: Ethanol + water soluble fraction (containing mainly soluble carbohydrates, amino acids, acids and phosphorylated intermediates), starch fraction, protein fraction and cell wall material.

As one would expect, also the photosynthetic ^{14}C-fixation is influenced by light quality in the same way, as shown for O_2-evolution. The rate of total fixation per cell decreases within 2 - 3 weeks in red light usually to about 1/5 to 1/7 of the initial value at the beginning of the red light treatment. In blue light, on the other hand, the rate of total ^{14}C incorporation increases slightly.

After two hours of photosynthesis most of the ^{14}C (70 - 85%) is present in the soluble fraction, than follows the starch fraction (5 - 15 %), cell wall material and only about 2 % of the ^{14}C fixed is incorporated into the protein fraction. As one should expect, the incorporation of ^{14}C in red light into all fractions decreases steadily with time. After 3 weeks in red light the rate of incorporation is only about 10 - 20 % of the initial value. Furthermore, the percentage distribution of ^{14}C on the different fractions is very similar at the beginning of the red light treatment and 3 weeks later. In blue light ^{14}C-incorporation into all fractions, except soluble fraction, increases with time. This result is not surprising since cells in blue light grow continuously. Stalk length increases from 5 mm up to about 30 mm during the course of the experiment and in addition some of the cells are forming caps.

Effect of light quality on the content of starch and soluble carbohydrates

There are still other differences between cells irradiated with red and blue light respectively. In Acetabularia mediterranea there are two fractions of polysaccharids:

starch and carbohydrates of the inulin-typeand in addition
the accompanying sugars of lower molecular weight, including fructose, saccharose, and glucose.

An examination of the carbohydrates revealed the following situation: In red light the amount of soluble sugars (fructose, glucose, sucrose, and fructosans) is fairly constant. In blue light, however, a steady increase
with time is observed (Fig. 3). The opposite situation is
found for the starch fraction. In red light the starch
content increases from 3,3 µg per cell at the beginning of
the experiment up to 13 µg after 3 weeks but only up to
6 µg in blue light in spite of the fact, that in blue
light the dry matter and protein content including chloroplastic protein have increased roughly by factor 3 compared with cells in red light.

The different starch contents of the chloroplasts can
also be demonstrated by means of electron microscopy.
Chloroplasts from cells grown in red light are crowded
with large starch granules, whereas chloroplasts from cells
grown in blue light have starch granules only scarcely and
if so very small ones.

This accumulation of starch in red light seems to be
not specific for Acetabularia. Similar results have been
obtained with Chlorella (8).

^{14}C-incorporation during the "induction period" in blue light, following red light

As we have seen (Fig. 2), the effect of red light on
photosynthesis is reversible. Transfering cells to continuous blue light, following red light treatment, results
in an increase of ^{14}C-fixation. Fig.4 demonstrates the
change in the rate of total fixation during this induction
period as a function of blue light treatment. The exposure
to blue light was started after 3 weeks in red light. The
following 8 hours in blue light do not remarkably influence the rate of total ^{14}C-fixation in the following 2 h in
white light, at light saturation. We have good evidence
from similar experiments, that there is a lag phase in the
order of about 8 - 10 hours indicating that something is
changing within the cell and very likely within the chloroplast itself to improve ^{14}C-fixation. The stimulation of

the fixation rate sets in between 10 h and 24 h and maximum fixation rates are usually obtained after 48 to 72 hours, followed by a more or less pronounced drop afterwards. This drop might be connected with an adaption to blue light condition, since cells grown in blue light only, have a lower fixation rate, similar to that after 144 h in blue light (Fig. 4).

As has been already mentioned up to 70 - 85 % of the ^{14}C fixed during 2 hours of photosynthesis is found in the soluble fraction. Therefore, the curve of total fixation reflects more or less the fixation into the soluble fraction. We will return to this fraction later on.

As opposed to the total fixation of ^{14}C, an increase of ^{14}C-incorporation into the protein fraction sets in earlier. Already after a period of 8 hours in blue light 5 times more ^{14}C is incorporated into protein (43.7 m µC/100 cells) than it is at the beginning of the blue light treatment (8.8 m µC/100 cells). We have good evidence from similar experiments that already after 2 hours in blue light there is a stimulation of incorporation in the order of 20 - 25 % into this fraction.

It seems therefore very likely, that a condition for the stimulation of the photosynthetic ^{14}C-fixation is the synthesis of special proteins taking place during the lag phase. This assumption is supported by experiments with inhibitors of protein synthesis. Puromycin, in a concentration of 30 µg/ml that inhibits the net synthesis of protein completely (9), prevents also completely the reinduction of photosynthesis (Fig. 5).

Since we are dealing with Acetabularia, the question arises inevitably whether this reinduction of photosynthesis in blue light is controlled by the nucleus. The answer is "no". Enucleated cells behave exactly so as do nucleated ones; i.e. in red light the rate of photosynthesis decreases and increases again in blue light even after 2 weeks in red light in the absence of the nucleus. Also in the presence of Actinomycin D in a concentration of 10 µg per ml that inhibits the transcription in the nucleus (10), an induction takes place in blue light (Fig. 5). The difference in the fixation rate of control cell (blue) and Actinomycin treated cell may be explained by a 40 % inhibition of photosynthesis by Actinomycin under these conditions. 30 µg Actinomycin D per ml prevents the stimulation of the ^{14}C-fixation almost completely. At this concentration

Actinomycin D inhibits photosynthesis and at the same time
strongly prevents the incorporation of ^{14}C into the protein
fraction, like Puromycin (30 µg/ml). These results roule
out the participation of a short living messenger formed
in the nucleus, but not with certainty the participation
of a messenger formed on the chloroplast DNA.

Besides stimulation of protein synthesis there are
some other changes in the metabolism during the induction
period in blue light. As already mentioned, cells grown
in red light are characterized by a high content of starch,
and a lower one in soluble carbohydrates (fructose, glucose,
sucrose, fructosan). Irradiation with blue light following
red light gives rise to a drastic reduction of starch (Fig.
6). Immediately, after the beginning of the treatment with
blue light, the starch content begins to decrease steadily
and reaches after 72 h about the value of cells grown in
continuous blue light. At the same time the rate of incorporation of ^{14}C into starch increases. Therefore, during
the induction period, a drastic increase in specific activity takes place from 12 m µC/mg starch at the beginning
of the blue light treatment up to about 500 m µC/mg starch
72 h later. The content of soluble carbohydrates, on the
other hand, increases steadily and reaches in accordance
with the starch fraction after 72 h the level of "blue
light" cells.

In order to get some information about the ^{14}C-incor-
poration into soluble carbohydrates, amino acids and acids,
including phosphorylated compounds, the soluble fraction
was further fractionated by means of ion exchange resins
into a basic, acidic and a neutral fraction.

It may be seen from fig. 7, that during the induction
phase the relative incorporation of ^{14}C into amino acids
and acids in the first instance decreases and increases
again after 48 h, whereas the relative incorporation into
the soluble sugar is firstly promoted and later on weake-
ned. This clearly shows, that during the induction period
not only a stimulation of ^{14}C incorporation takes place,
but also some shifts in the metabolic pattern.

A chromatographic analysis of the sugar fraction
(neutral subfraction of the soluble fraction) shows, that
during the pretreatment with red light the percentage of
^{14}C fixed into the fructosan compounds with higher molecular weights (inulin) is decreasing. Fig. 8 (0 h) shows the

situation after 3 weeks in red light. 35 % of ^{14}C of the
neutral fraction is present in fructose, 18 % in glucose,
39 % in sucrose, and only 8 % in inulin. During the following radiation with blue light the proportion of ^{14}C in
fructose, sucrose, and glucose decreases steadily with
time and increases in the inulin. Data on the quantitative
changes in the concentration of the individual sugars are
not available at the moment. Particularly it has to be
proved, whether the observed increase in the amount of soluble carbohydrates (Fig. 6) is mainly due to inulin.

Final remarks

This is a rough picture of our present knowledge on
the effect of red and blue light on the metabolism of
Acetabularia. It is without any doubt, that the light
quality has a profound influence on photosynthesis (and
consequently on growth), carbohydrate metabolism and synthesis of protein, starch and cell wall material. This
multiple influence on different reactions makes it impossible to give at present a general picture on the effect
of blue and red light, respectively.
Speaking about the influence of red and blue light
on photosynthesis of Acetabularia we have to mention another effect of blue light on the metabolism of algae i.e.
the stimulation of respiration, especially studied in
Chlorella (10). It seems very likely, that there are some
connection between both phenomena. For example, the action
spetra of both reactions are quite similar (7, 14). Furthermore, the degradation of starch in blue light suggests,
that a stimulation of respiration might be involved in the
blue light dependent enhancement of photosynthesis in
Acetabularia. It could be possible, that the degradation
products of starch are being used as substrates for the
respiration and in this way giving rise to the synthesis
of carbon skeleton for amino acids formation which are
needed for the synthesis of protein involved in the induction of photosynthesis.
The antagonistic effect of red and blue light on
the content of starch and soluble carbohydrates suggests
another possibility that might explain the light effects,
at least in part. As we have seen, in red light the

accumulation of starch is promoted. At the same time the content of soluble sugars, including fructosan is relatively low. In blue light, on the other hand, the content of soluble sugars and fructosans increases and the starch content decreases. Starch is localized in the chloroplasts and probably most of the soluble sugars and the fructosans in the cytoplasm. These facts could be an indication that light quality has an effect on chloroplast permeability. It might be possible, that in red light the membrane of the chloroplast gets increasingly impermeable for the products of photosynthesis so favouring the synthesis of starch in the chloroplast, thus reducing the content of soluble sugars and fructosans in the cytoplasm. Blue light, on the other hand, would remove this barrier.

One might speculate further that the reduction of the rate of photosynthesis has a similar reason and is only due to a barrier for CO_2 entrance into the chloroplast, formed in red light. However, the reduction of Hill activity in red light contradicts this possibility. It is more likely, that red light acts actively or passively on the membran system of the chloroplast.

Which of these possibilities are realized is, at present, unknown.

Acknowledgements

The author wish to thank the Deutsche Forschungsgemeinschaft for supporting these investigations. Thanks are also due to Mrs. Maass for valuable technical assistance.

References

1. K. Beth, Z.Naturforschg. 8b, 334 (1953);
                            10b, 267 (1955).
2. Terborgh and K.V. Thimann, Planta 63, 83 (1964);
   Planta 64, 241 (1965).
3. H. Mohr, Planta 47, 127 (1956).
4. G. Richter, Naturwiss. 49, 238 (1962).
5. H. Clauss, Naturwiss. 50, 719 (1963);
   Protoplasma 65, 49 (1968).

6. J. Terborgh, Nature 207, 1360 (1965).
7. J. Terborgh, Plant Physiol. 41, 1401 (1966).
8. U. Schael and H. Clauss, Planta 78, 98 (1968).
9. H. Clauss, unpublished results.
10. A. Pirson, personal communication.
11. K. Zetsche, Z.Naturforschg. 21b, 88 (1966).
12. K. Zetsche, Z.Naturforschg. 19b, 751 (1964).
13. W. Kowallik and H. Gaffron, Planta 69, 92 (1966).
14. W. Kowallik, Plant Physiol. 42, 672 (1967).

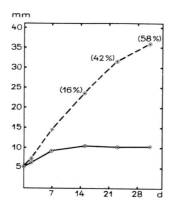

Fig. 1
Growth of Acetabularia mediterranea cells in red and blue
light. Cell with a stalk length of 30 - 35 mm were cut
down to 5 mm and transfered to red and blue light 24 h
later. ⊙————⊙ red light, ⊙————⊙ blue light.
Light conditions: continuous light, 4000 erg cm^{-2}sec^{-1}.
Abscissa: days. Ordinate: stalk length in mm.
Numbers (%) = cells with cap in percentage.

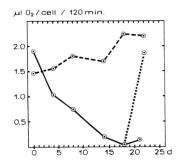

μl O$_2$/cell / 120 min.

Fig. 2
Net photosynthesis of <u>Acetabularia mediterranea</u> in red
and blue light. Cells with a stalk length of 30 - 35 mm
were cut down to 20 mm and transfered to red and blue
light, respectively. Part of the cells was transfered
from red to blue light after 19 days. After various periods of time cells were allowed to photosynthate for
2 hours under the same light condition. O$_2$ evolution was
determined electrochemically (8).

   ⊙————⊙ red light, ⊙————⊙   blue light,
   ⊙ ...... ⊙ 18 d red light ————➔ blue light.
Abscissa: days. Ordinate: Net photosynthesis
μl O$_2$ per cell per 120 min. Light intensity 4000 erg.
cm^{-2}sec^{-1}.

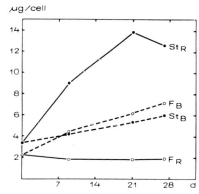

μg/cell

Fig. 3
Quantitative changes of starch and soluble carbohydrates
in cells of <u>Acetabularia mediterranea</u> in red and blue
light. Cell material and light conditions as in figure 1.
Cells in blue light: ●— — — —● starch (St$_B$),
o — — — —o soluble carbohydrates (F$_B$).
Cells in red light: ●————● starch (St$_R$),
o————o soluble carbohydrates (F$_R$).
Abscissa: days. Ordinate: μg per cell.

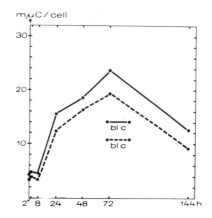

Fig. 4

Changes in the rate of photosynthesis in <u>Acetabularia</u>
<u>mediterranea</u> during the "induction period" in blue light,
following red light treatment. Cell material as in fig. 1.
Cells were kept for 3 weeks in continuous red light and
then transfered to continuous blue light. After various
periods of time in blue light, cells were allowed to photosynthate for 2 hours in white light at light saturation
($\sim$ 800 ftc) in the presence of $NaH^{14}CO_3$.
●————● total fixation, ●－－－－● fixation in the
(ethanol + water) soluble fraction. bl c = fixation rate
of cells in continuous blue light.
Abscissa: time in blue light. Ordinate: fixation rate in
m µC/cell/per 2 h.

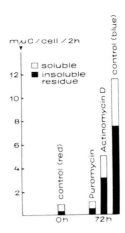

Fig. 5
Effect of Puromycin and Actinomycin D on the induction of
photosynthesis in blue light after pretreatment with red
light. Cell material as in fig. 1. After 3 weeks in red
light the algae were transfered to blue light (except control red) and kept in Puromycin (30 µg/ml), Actinomycin D
(10 µg/ml) and without any addition (control blue). After
72 hours cells were allowed to photosynthate for 2 h in
$NaH^{14}CO_3$ containing medium in the absence of any inhibitor.
Light condition: 4000 erg $cm^{-2}sec^{-1}$, continuous light.
Ordinate: incorporation rate of ^{14}C in m µC.

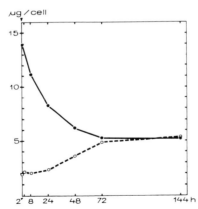

Fig. 6
Quantitative changes in starch and soluble sugars in blue
light after red light pretreatment. Cell material and
light conditions as in fig. 1. Cells were pretreated with
red light for 3 weeks and then transfered to blue light.
●————● starch, o—————o soluble carbohydrates.
Abscissa: hours in blue light. Ordinate: µg per cell.

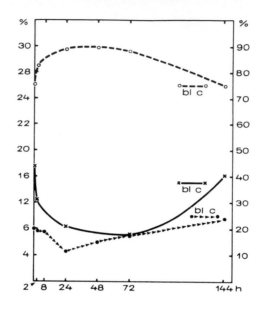

Fig. 7
Percentage distribution of ^{14}C incorporated into the soluble fraction on soluble carbohydrate, amino acids and acids, including phosphorylated intermediates during the "induction period". Cell material and light conditions as in fig. 6.
o – – – – o soluble carbohydrates. x ———— x amino acids,
● ► ► ► ● acid + phosphorylated compounds.
Abscissa: hours in blue light. Ordinate: percentage incorporation. Left: for amino acids and acids, right: for soluble carbohydrates.

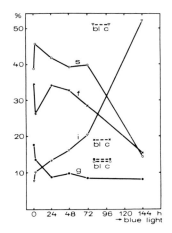

Fig. 8
Percentage distribution of ^{14}C on the individual sugars of
the soluble fraction during the "individual period". Cell
material and light conditions as in fig. 6. x ———x
fructose, ●———● glucose, o ———o sucrose,
▽———▽ higher polymer fructosan ("inulin"). Abscissa:
hours in blue light. Ordinate: percentage.

191

JUNE 20 (MOL)
MORNING SESSION

Chairman: Cyrille H. V. Sironval

PHOTOSYNTHESIS IN CHLOROPLASTS ISOLATED FROM
ACETABULARIA MEDITERRANEA

David C. Shephard

Department of Anatomy
Case Western Reserve University
Cleveland, Ohio

Abstract

Chloroplasts isolated from Acetabularia by low
speed centrifugation in mannitol media appear to carry out
complete photosynthesis. Measurements using an oxygen
electrode show:
1. These chloroplasts appear to have an endogenous dark
   respiration that does not respond to mitochondrial substrates or inhibitors.
2. In light and in the presence of reducible carbon compounds oxygen is evolved.
3. ADP, NADP and ferridoxin when added to the medium will
   not support oxygen evolution.
4. Calvin cycle intermediates do not increase the oxygen
   evolution rate in the presence of saturating bicarbonate.
5. The photosynthetic rate approaches that seen in the
   intact cell when compared per mg chlorophyll.

Factors in the isolation and assay procedures are discussed
and criteria for evaluating the chloroplast fraction are
proposed.

Introduction

Chloroplasts isolated from Acetabularia mediterranea carry out normal photosynthesis at high rates for ex-
tended periods of time (1). Experiments using ^{14}C have

195

demonstrated that the pattern of carbon intermediates is the same as seen in vivo (1, 2). This chloroplast fraction also has an endogenous CO_2 evolution with the characteristics of photorespiration and dark respiration (3). Thus these chloroplasts isolated from Acetabularia appear to be unsurpassed by any of the photosynthetically active fractions isolated recently by several other laboratories (4,5,6,7,8) and they should provide excellent material for studies of a variety of chloroplast activities.

The isolation and assay procedures for these chloroplasts were originally developed using a polarographic oxygen electrode. Considerable data on the behavior of the fraction were obtained with this rapid and convenient assay system. These data relate to the handling of the chloroplasts, the composition of the isolation media, the optimum assay conditions and the systems responsible for both the oxygen consumption and oxygen evolution. Moreover these assays confirm dramatically the observations that intact chloroplasts retain the critical intermediates and cofactors required for maximal photosynthetic rates (6) and that the photosystems are tightly coupled to carbon fixation as has been suggested by Walker and Hill (5).

Materials and Methods

Cells

The cells used were from stocks of Acetabularia mediterranea grown in my laboratory. They had been propagated for several generations in a chemically defined medium at 22°-24°C with a 12 hr on 12 hr off light cycle using 200 fc of flourescent lighting. The procedures for growing and handling the cells have been described in detail (9); however the cells used in these experiments were not axenic. The chloroplast fraction was obtained from cells in the exponential phase of growth (10); usually they were between 1.5 and 2.0 cm in length. Occasionally experiments were carried out with larger cells but all those with caps were eliminated. The isolation procedure was begun by putting the cells on ice at the same time of day (4 hrs after lights on) to avoid any problems with circadian rhythms.

Chloroplast Isolation

Outlines of schemes for isolating these chloroplasts have been presented previously (1,3). Figure 1 presents a similar scheme. There is nothing very unusual in these procedures except the scissor mincing which cuts each cell into numerous small fragments from which the cytoplasm leaks spontaneously. Although the procedures work well, several aspects are subject to improvement or should be tested in more detail. The isolation media can almost certainly be improved. Mannitol has two drawbacks: it is probably a metabolite for marine organisms, and isosmolar (to sea water) amounts will not remain in solution at $0°C$. TES buffer (11) is probably completely satisfactory, and its use at 0.1 M in the "H" medium is necessary to neutralize the vacuolar acidity. The EDTA, BSA and DTT are all beneficial but their concentrations have not been thoroughly evaluated. Ascorbate or isoascorbate have no apparent effect. Of the salts in the assay medium, it is likely that the orthophosphate should be replaced by pyrophosphate and that Ca^{++}, Mn^{++}, NO_3^- and SO_4^- should be represented.

The maximum centrifugal force that can be used depends on the density and viscosity of the medium. If too much force is applied under unsuitable conditions starch grains are ripped out of the chloroplasts and sediment as a whitish layer at the bottom of the pellet. The presence of such a layer signifies chloroplast damage and will be seen if more than 500 x g is applied in "W" medium. When dextran or Ficoll is used to increase the density or viscosity of the medium the damage will occur at lower centrifugal forces. Sucrose appears to enter the chloroplast so readily as to be of little value in increasing medium density. Bottom layers (pads) of 20% dextran or Ficoll in W will usually not be entered by the chloroplasts at 350 x g or less and are useful at times. Even at these low forces most of the chloroplasts may be sedimented in 20 minutes. It is necessary to have close control of the centrifuge at low speeds and to keep track of the radius at various levels in the tubes. The fractionation scheme given in Figure 1 yields only slightly cleaner chloroplasts than repeated differential sedimentations at 350 x g.

A major flaw in the isolation procedure is that during the scissor mincing of the cells, droplets of cytoplasm are formed containing several organelles plus associated cytoplasm enclosed in a membrane (tonoplast/plasmalemma). These droplets are difficult to disrupt during the subsequent operations at least without doing serious damage to the chloroplasts. Several strokes with a Dounce homogenizer serve to break the larger ones but are not adequate to disrupt all of them. If only the smaller chloroplasts are needed, a 3 min, 100 x g pellet can be discarded; it will contain most of these droplets along with the amyloplasts and larger chloroplasts. Another method of reducing the frequency of droplets, and other debris as well, is to pass the suspension through a Millipore filter type NC (nylon, 14 μ pore). Gentle pressure rather than vacuum should be used and smaller pore filters will not pass the chloroplasts undamaged.

The Oxygen Electrode

Clark type oxygen electrodes (12) manufactured by the Yellow Springs Instrument Co. Yellow Springs, Ohio were used throughout with 1 mil (0.001 inch) Teflon membranes. A dual channel amplifier and polarization voltage supply was designed and built by an associate : David Rosner. A timing mechanism and a low noise relay feeds the signal from the two channels alternately to a potentiometric chart recorder. The zeros and sensitivities of the channels can be adjusted independently on the chart. Zero and 100% points were set with circulating dry nitrogen and air respectively. Assays were usually made in 3 ml total volume and continuous rapid stirring of the mixture was required. Additions to the reaction mixture were made with a Hamilton syringe in aliquots of 0.03 ml (1% of the usual volume). The entire assay chamber was immersed in a 20 gallon, temperature controlled aquarium. A 150 W incandescent spot light at the side was used for illumination and resulted in little or no heating of the sample in the circulating water of the aquarium. The temperature for all measurements was 24°C, and for all calculations it has been assumed that 5 μl of oxygen will be dissolved in 1 ml of A medium in equilibrum with air at 24°C. Chlorophyll determinations were made on an 80% acetone extract of the chloroplast pellet by the method of Arnon (13).

When A medium was to be deoxygenated or decarbonated, purified nitrogen was passed through an Ascarite
column then rehumidified and bubbled through the medium
for at least 30 min. It was not possible to treat the
chloroplasts so harshly. The chloroplast pellet was suspended in 0.5 ml of A medium containing 1-3 mg of carbonic
anhydrase and placed in a closed container as a shallow
layer. A magnetic stirrer was added and moist, CO_2 free
nitrogen was passed over the suspension for 10 min or more.
A few minutes of illumination helps to remove the last traces of CO_2 from the chloroplast sample. A nitrogen flushed
syringe was used to transfer medium and chloroplasts to
the nitrogen filled assay chamber. With practice it was
possible to load the chamber so that the chloroplasts
could carry out neither photosynthesis nor respiration until either bicarbonate or oxygen had been added. The carbonic anhydrase has no effect on the rates or products of
photosynthesis (3).

Results

When washed, isolated chloroplasts in A medium are
simply placed in the oxygen electrode chamber an oxygen
exchange such as shown in Figure 2 can be seen. In darkness the preparation consumes oxygen at a rate of approximately 5 µl/min/mg chlorophyll. When the preparation is
brightly illuminated there is an almost immediate evolution of oxygen and a maximum rate of approximately 20
µl/min/mg chlorophyll (60 micromoles/hr/mg chlorophyll) is
achieved within 30 sec to 1 min. The preparation will continue to perform in this manner for a number of hours despite continuous stirring (Figure 2 represents almost 2
hours). The rates of oxygen evolution and consumption remain nearly constant from air levels of oxygen to 10% of
this level. The sturdiness and consistency of these chloroplasts are truly amazing.

Attempts were made to answer the following questions
with this chloroplast fraction.
1. What organelle or enzyme system is responsible for the
    dark oxygen consumption or respiration?
2. Does the oxygen evolution in the light represent com-
    plete photosynthesis or merely photosystem II activi-
    ty?

199

3. What aspects of preparatory and assay procedure maximize the rates of oxygen exchange and how do the maximum rates compare with the intact cell rates?

Oxygen consumption

It was initialy assumed that mitochondrial contamination of the chloroplast fraction was responsible for the respiration; therefore attempts were made to enhance the oxygen consumption rate by the addition of mitochondrial substrates. Figure 3 shows the absence of any effect following the addition of succinate, ADP, then malate and finally by the addition of the mitochondrial inhibitor--amytal. The apparent slight effect of the amytal is due to the low oxygen tension not the drug. Subsequent efforts failed to demonstrate any enhancement of the rate of oxygen consumption by the addition of substrate amounts of NADH (0.1mM), pyruvate (1 mM), citrate (1 mM) or alpha-ketoglutarate (1 m M), nor any reduction in rate by inhibitory concentrations of cyanide (0.1mM), iodoacetate (1 mM), arsenite (10 μM) or malonate (10 mM). In all cases the recorder traces were examined for at least 10 min after the additions. Although longer term treatments or preincubations were not preformed, it seemed unlikely that the oxygen consumption was due to mitochondrial contamination. Moreover, an easily measurable NAD malic dehydrogenase activity (assay of Ochoa, 14) sedimented readily from the chloroplast supernatants and was reduced in the chloroplast fraction progressively during the washes. The oxygen consumption of the chloroplast fraction was not diminished by washing.

Although bacteria should have responded to some of the mitochondrial substrates, further tests for contamination by microorganisms seemed in order. No effect was apparent after the addition of glucose, but in the presence of 0.6M mannitol this was not too surprising. Attempts were made to replace the mannitol in the A medium with polyethylene glycol (average molecular weight 400). The chloroplasts were not very long lived in this medium, but they had a respectable oxygen consumption. As in normal medium respiration was not enhanced by the addition of various substrates; thus the respiration must occur at the expense of some substrate in the fraction, possibly an internal storage product such as starch.

At this point it seemed most likely that the oxygen consumption was an inherent property of the chloroplasts themselves. Therefore an attempt was made to stimulate the respiratory rate with substrate amounts (1 mM) of several likely photosynthetic products: 3-phosphoglycerate, glycolate and glyoxylate. No effect was seen, nor was any inhibition seen following the addition of α-hydroxy-2-pyridinemethanesulfanate-- an inhibitor of photorespiration (15). Thus on the basis of the oxygen exchange measurements it was impossible to reach any definite conclusions concerning the systems involved in the oxygen consumption of the chloroplast fraction except that respiration seemed to be a property of the chloroplasts themselves rather than of a contaminant of the fraction. Measurements of carbon exchange support this observation (3).

Oxygen evolution

The next important question -- does the oxygen evolution represent photosynthesis or simply photosystem II activity -- can be asked of the oxygen measurements by determining what compounds act as the final electron and proton acceptors. By the simple expedient of driving the bicarbonate (CO_2) content of the medium down to zero it could be shown that carbon was acting as the acceptor; in other words that the system carried out carbon reduction and in all likelihood -- complete photosynthesis. Figure 4 presents these data and also a determination of the saturating bicarbonate concentration at the usual pH and temperature of the A medium. This figure also shows that a minute amount of detergent is sufficient to destroy the photosynthetic activity of the chloroplasts.

Attempts were made to determine whether exogenously supplied ADP, NADP or ferridoxin could replace bicarbonate in supporting oxygen evolution. As shown in Figure 5 they could not. Other experiments indicated that these compounds also did not enhance the rate of oxygen evolution when HCO_3^- was present. Thus the photosystems appear to be tightly coupled to carbon fixation probably because of the highly selective nature of the chloroplast membrane. Exogenously supplied proton and electron acceptors do not gain access (see 16); therefore carbon must be reduced to regenerate these compounds in the internal pool of the chloroplast.

Maximizing the Rate of Oxygen Evolution

It was desirable to determine the saturating conditions for light and carbon dioxide. The unreasonable partial pressure of 2.5 mm CO_2 is in equilibrum with the 1 mM saturating level of HCO_3^- at pH 7.5 and 24°C. Normal sea water (pH 8.1) however, also contains approximately 1 mM HCO_3^- ; thus it appears that HCO_3^- not CO_2 is the form of carbon used by these chloroplasts or at least it is the form transported across the membranes. Because of the interrelationship of pH, HCO_3^- and CO_2 there are also problems in determining a pH optimum. Using a modified chamber incorporating both a pH electrode and the oxygen probe a broad optimum between pH 7 and pH 8 was found. Irreversible losses in activity occurred below pH 6.8 and above pH 8.2. The 1 mM saturating level of HCO_3^- held over this entire range, or in other words photosynthesis saturated at a similar rate over a range of pH dependant CO_2 concentrations from 10 mm P CO_2 at pH 6.8 to 0.3 mm $P CO_2$ at pH 8.2 (see discussion in 3).

Light saturation is easier to determine but it, of course, depends on the concentration of chloroplasts in the assay medium and the geometry of the assay chamber. For the system used, with typically 100 μg chlorophyll in 3 ml of medium, in a chamber 2 cm in diameter , illuminated from the side with incandescent light, oxygen evolution was saturated at 20 mW/cm^2 (approximately 2000 fc).

No attempt has been made to determine a temperature optimum. The temperature used was the same at which the cells were grown.

Since several laboratories had reported that the rate of photosynthesis in isolated chloroplasts was increased by the addition of Calvin cycle intermediates (4), ribose-5-phosphate, fructose-1,6- diphosphate and 3-phosphoglycerate (PGA) were added to Acetabularia chloroplasts. The sugar phosphates did not increase the rate of oxygen evolution indicating an impermeable membrane and probably an adequate internal concentration. The PGA – a reducible carbon source – supported oxygen evolution and thus was able to penetrate the membrane readily (see 6). As seen in Figure 6 the rate of oxygen evolution supported by the

PGA was less than maximum, and was increased by the addition of bicarbonate. In the presence of saturating bicarbonate the addition of PGA had no stimulatory effect on oxygen evolution. These observations strongly suggest that the chloroplasts are intact and that all necessary components are retained during the process of isolation.

Since the activity of the isolated chloroplasts seemed so nearly normal a comparison of oxygen evolution by intact cells and isolated chloroplasts was made. The data are shown in Figure 7. The cells were in their normal medium, partially desoxygenated, and adjusted to pH 7.5, while the chloroplasts were in A medium at pH 7.5. Repeated bicarbonate additions were made to assure the saturation of both systems and light was above the saturation level. Subsequent to the measurements the chlorophyll in each sample was determined. The rate of oxygen evolution by the cells was expected to be as high as or possibly higher that in normal culture conditions where less light and bicarbonate are available inside the closed culture bottles. The observed (Fig.7) intact cell rate of 26 μl/min/mg chlorophyll (about 70 μMole/hour per mg chlorophyll) is rather low compared to other green plants, but then Acetabularia has a low growth rate too. The isolated chloroplasts evolved oxygen 18 μl/min/mg chlorophyll – more than two thirds of the intact cell rate. These chloroplasts were less active than usual and rates in excess of 20 μl/min/mg chlorophyll (80% of the intact cell rate) are frequently observed. These figures for photosynthetic oxygen evolution, although a bit low, are entirely comparable to those for carbon fixation obtained by entirely different means and reported elsewhere (3). Few other chloroplast isolates have been reported to obtain nearly 75% of the intact cell photosynthetic rate and maintain photosynthesis for long periods of time (4,5,6,7,8).

Discussion

The main purpose in studying isolated chloroplasts is to determine the metabolic pattern intrinsic to the chloroplast and the pathways by which this pattern interacts with that of the rest of the cell. Both the metabolic pattern and the controlled transfer of metabolites or other materials depend on chloroplast structure; hence the current interest in "intact" isolated chloroplasts. The criteria for intactness, however, are not very clear. Moreover, to yield the information desired the chloroplasts must be, not only intact, but also free from contamination by other structures capable of distorting the metabolic pattern seen, and criteria are very scarce here. Phase microscopy and electron microscopy showing a complete outer membrane have been used as criteria for intactness by Leech (17) who has also used the presence and absence of certain enzymes to monitor the contamination by mitochondria. Although it seems logical to monitor structure by morphological means and to search for contaminants by means of characteristic chemical constituents; in practice the reverse procedure may give more reliable results.

Acetabularia chloroplasts provide a case in point. If they are isolated in high molarity salt solutions or in the presence of excess orthophosphate they are quite intact by Leech's criteria but they are photosynthetically inactive. On the other hand physiologically active chloroplasts may lose all semblance of intactness during processing for the electron microscope. In both cases the intactness is better measured by physiological activity. On the other hand, phase and electron microscopy of Acetabularia chloroplast fractions reveal contamination by mitochondria and other cytoplasmic constituents as well as bacteria; however, measurements of respiratory, activity attributable to mitochondria and bacteria have not suggested the presence of significant contamination.

The problem with a morphological definition of intactness is that functional intactness is desired and it is impossible to specify the morphology in sufficient detail to be certain of physiological state. The physiological investigation of the presence of contaminants sufferes from a similar lack of complete knowledge. One can not be certain that a particular activity of a suspected contaminant will be measurable or that the activity might not also be endogenous to the structure being isolated. On the basis of these arguments it seems reasonable to establish the following criteria for the intactness and freedom from contamination of chloroplast fractions. 1) Intactness: Chloroplasts are intact when in a minimally complex isolation medium they exhibit the characteristic photosynthetic activities at the maximum predictable rate; i.e. that seen in the intact cell from which they were isolated. It is, of course, possible that this rate might be exceeded when the chloroplast is freed from the constraints of the rest of the cell. 2) Contamination: The fraction is contaminated if there is anything besides chloroplasts visible in it. The examination should really use both phase and Electron microscopy.

The Acetabularia chloroplast fraction can be evaluated by these criteria. It is at least as intact as any previously reported fraction and little more improvement is necessary to reach the intact cell rate of photosynthesis. The level of contamination, however, is definitely worse than that seen in other plants. The reasons for this are as follows: First Acetabularia is typically grown in contaminated fluid cultures and bacteria will be found in the isolated chloroplast pellets, often in large numbers. Second, the easy rupture of the cell wall that may be largely responsible for chloroplast intactness also facilitates for formation of the cytoplasmic droplets containing mitochondria and other materials having the size and density to sediment in the chloroplast fraction.

Thus, isolated Acetabularia chloroplasts which seem so desirable for studying photosynthetic processes that are thought to be exclusive plastid activities may make rather poor subjects for the study of suspected chloroplast functions that are also actively carried out in other parts of the cytoplasm or in contaminating microorganisms. Growth of Acetabularia in axenic culture and some improvements in isolation technique are all that are needed to make these chloroplast truly superb.

Acknowledgements

The support of the National Science Foundation (GB 5210) is appreciated. The oxygen electrode apparatus was constructed with a General Research Support Grant from Western Reserve University.

References

1. D.C. Shephard, W.B. Levin and R.G.S. Bidwell, Biochem. Biophys. Res. Commun. 32, 413, (1968).
2. R.G.S. Bidwell, W.B. Levin and D.C. Shephard, Plant Physiol. in press.
3. R.G.S. Bidwell, W.B. Levin and D.C. Shephard, Plant Physiol. 44, 946, (1969).
4. R. G. Jensen and J.A. Bassham, Biochim. Biophys. Acta 153, 219, (1968).
5. D.A. Walker and R. Hill, Biochim. Biophys. Acta 131, 330, (1967).
6. J. M. Robinson and C.R. Stocking, Plant Physiol. 43, 1597, (1968).
7. M. Gibbs, E.S. Bamberger, P.W. Ellyard and R.G. Everson, in "Biochemistry of the Chloroplasts" vol.2, p. 3, T.W. Goodwin, ed., Academic Press N.Y. (1966).
8. D. I. Arnon, in "Biochemistry of the Chloroplasts" vol. 2, p. 461, T. W. Goodwin, ed., Academic Press, N.Y. (1966).
9. D. C. Shephard, in "Methods in Cell Physiology" vol. 4, D. Prescott, ed. in press, Academic Press, N.Y.
10. D. C. Shephard, Exp. Cell Res. 37, 93, (1965).
11. N. E. Good, G. D. Winget, W. Winter, T.N. Connolly, S. Izawa and R. M. M. Singh, Biochemistry 5, 467, (1966).
12. R. W. Estabrook, in "Methods in Enzymology" vol. X, p.41, R. W. Estabrook and M.E. Pullman eds. Academic Press, N.Y. (1967).
13. D. I. Arnon, Plant Physiol. 24, 1, (1949).
14. S. Ochoa, in "Methods in Enzymology" vol. I, p. 735, S.P. Colowick and N.O. Kaplan eds. Academic Press, N.Y. (1955).
15. I. Zelitch, J. Biol. Chem. 224, 251, (1957).
16. H. Strotmann and S. Berger, Biochem. Biophys. Res. Commun. 35, 20, (1968).
17. R. M. Leech, in "Biochemistry of the Chloroplasts" vol. 1. p. 65, T. W. Goodwin ed., Academic Press, N.Y. (1966).

Mince 3 g of cells (about 300, 2 cm cells) in 6 ml of H medium.
Strain the resulting slurry through 270 mesh bolting nylon.
Rinse the debris with 15 ml of W medium. All operations are
carried out on ice.

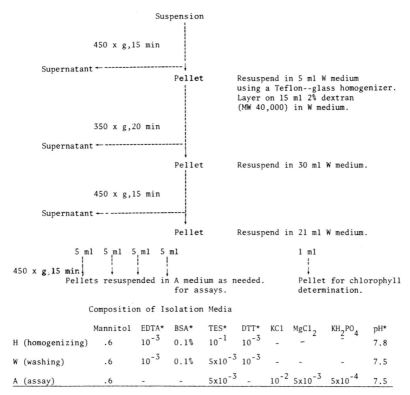

Composition of Isolation Media

	Mannitol	EDTA*	BSA*	TES*	DTT*	KCl	MgCl$_2$	KH$_2$PO$_4$	pH*
H (homogenizing)	.6	10^{-3}	0.1%	10^{-1}	10^{-3}	-	-		7.8
W (washing)	.6	10^{-3}	0.1%	5×10^{-3}	10^{-3}	-	-	-	7.5
A (assay)	.6	-	-	5×10^{-3}	-	10^{-2}	5×10^{-3}	5×10^{-4}	7.5

* EDTA=disodium ethylenediaminetetraacetate, BSA= bovine serum albumin,
  TES= n-tris (hydroxymethyl) methyl-2-aminoethanesulfonic acid,
  DTT= dithiothreitol. pH adjusted with KOH.

Figure 1. Fractionation

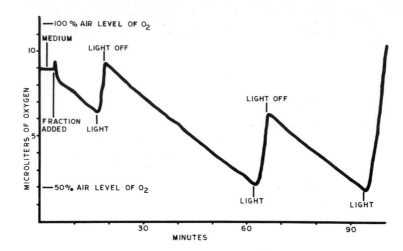

Figure 2.   The Oxygen Exchange of the Chloroplast Fraction.
The ordinate is adjusted on the chart to represent 0-100% of the air saturation level of
oxygen. This can be translated to microliters
of dissolved O_2: 20%= 1 µl O_2/ml assay medium.
A downward slope represents a consumption of
oxygen and a rising slope, an evolution. On the
original chart the time scale was such that
events that lasted only a few seconds could be
followed.

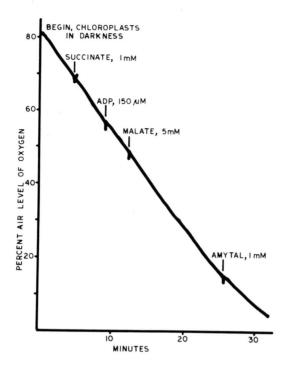

Figure 3. Oxygen Consumption by the Chloroplast Fraction.
The substrates and inhibitors are added until
they reach the stated concentration in the assay mixture.

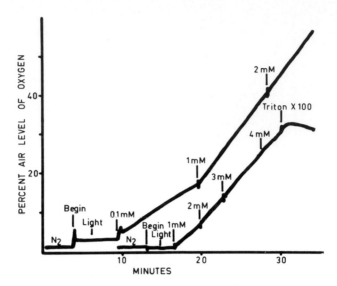

Figure 4.   Bicarbonate Dependent Oxygen Evolution. The
assay mixture was completely deoxygenated and
decarbonated for these measurements. The probe
was in nitrogen above the assay mixture and
was lowered into the mixture to begin. No oxygen exchange could be measured before or after
the light was turned on until bicarbonate was
added. The rate of oxygen evolution saturated
at between 1 and 2 mM bicarbonate. The addition
of 0.01% Triton X-100 caused an immediate ces-
sation of oxygen evolution.

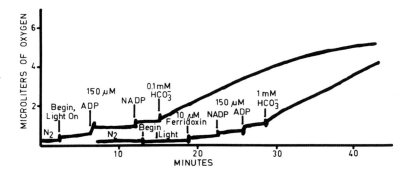

Figure 5. Lack of Dissociable Photosystem Activity. Conditions were as in Figure 4. The additions themselves introduce a small amount of dissolved oxygen and possibly CO_2. This accounts for the rise in O_2 level and a barely measurable rate of oxygen evolution. The substrates themselves, with the exception of HCO_3^-, do not support any measurable oxygen evolution.

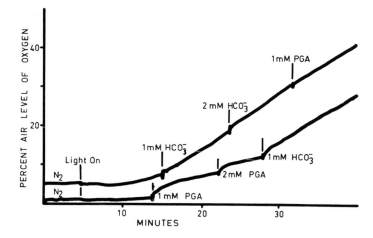

Figure 6. Phosphoglycerate as a Substrate. This is a dual channel simultaneous trace. Except for the additions the two channels are identical. Note that the final rates are parallel. The oxygen evolution supported by 3 phosphoglycerate (PGA) can be increased by the addition of bicarbonate but not the reverse.

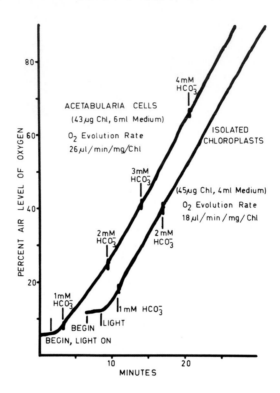

Figure 7.   Isolated Chloroplasts and Whole Cells.
The chloroplasts evolve oxygen at two thirds
the rate of the whole cells on a per mg chlorophyll (Chl) basis.

TEMPORAL REGULATION IN ACETABULARIA

Thérèse Vanden Driessche

Laboratoire de Morphologie Animale,
Université Libre de Bruxelles,
Brussels, Belgium.

Abstract

The various rhythms of Acetabularia mediterranea are described (with regard to the rhythm in polysaccharide content, new information concerning the nature of the reserve material is reported). The possible interdependence of certain oscillations is discussed. Clearly, Acetabularia is endowed with an elaborated temporal morphology.

All the overt processes seem to be embodied by proteins, possibly allosteric.

The effects of the inhibitors of transcription and translation, the effects of anucleation and grafting show that the nucleus controls the basic mechanism of rhythmicity by means of long-lived RNAs.

The prevalent ideas about circadian rhythmicity are summarized and the general relevance of these findings is discussed.

Introduction

About half a century ago, it must have been an extraordinary experience to find out that each function has a precise intracellular localization and that the operation of many of them requires an intact structure. Nowadays we are discovering that a fourth dimension has to be taken into account : time.

The normal development of an organism is strictly

dependent on a precise sequence of events. In higher plants, a long series of sequentional events leads to the formation of a mature plant, able to reproduce. In the case of Acetabularia, it has been demonstrated by Brachet (1) that any perturbation in the normal sequence of transcription and translation - for example as a result of impaired proteosynthesis due to puromycin - interfers with the normal formation of reproductive caps.

Clauss (2) and Terborgh (3,4) have shown how great the influences of the quality and the quantity of light are on growth and morphogenesis in Acetabularia. However, next to nothing is known about the requirements and mechanisms through which the alga enters the reproductive phase or germinates. Cytoplasmic factors must be implicated, since it is well known that Acetabularia cells can be maintained in the vegetative state, simply by repeatedly severing the apex.

In other species, though many details remain to be clarified, much indirect evidence suggests that flowering can occur only if certain conditions are fulfilled. The main factor for inducing flowering in many higher plants is the ratio between the light and the dark periods of a 24 h cycle (5, 6, 7, 8). It is not known whether it influences the cycle of Acetabularia ; this is one of the numerous open problems that have to be solved.

Not only does the synthesis of certain substances take place only during a limited period of the developmental processes, but the capacity or intensity of a number of functions vary with the time of the day. These oscillations in the rate of a function are often measured as changes in the content of a product. Temporal morphology is the term that Halberg (9) has recently coined for the description of the time functions, the main aspect being the circadian rhythmicity.

In this paper, the various circadian rhythms of Acetabularia will be described. Their endogenous nature has been checked. No attempt, however, has been made up to now to elucidate the possible changes in phase-relationships of the different circadian functions when the cells are transferred from L:D to constant conditions, either L:L or D:D.[x]

[x]Abbreviations: L: D, light-dark culture conditions; the durations of the respective light and dark periods are indicated by the following figures. L period of illumination; D period of darkness; LL, DD, continuous light or dark.

Two new circadian rhythms will be described: one in ATP
content, as determined with E.Schram, and one in fructose
incorporation, studied with S. Bonotto. About the variation in polysaccharide content, the results recently obtained as to the nature of the carbohydrates of the sedimentable fraction will be briefly summarized.

The oscillation of certain functions might be merely
the consequence of the oscillation of other functions:
the interdependence of the various rhythms will be discussed.

A scheme will be presented, which summarizes the present biochemical evidence regarding temporal regulation
in Acetabularia.

Finally, the general models tentatively explaining the
mechanism of circadian rhythmicity will be discussed and
some new ideas suggested.

The temporal morphology of Acetabularia

The circadian rhythms are graphically represented in
time-maps, which allow easy comparison between the phases.
In these maps, the observed values are calculated as relative value, i.e. as percent of the mean of the day, and
plotted against time.

Rhythm in RNA synthesis

This rhythm is measured by the incorporation of ^{3}H-
uridine in the acid-insoluble fraction (10) (fig.1). The
maximum occurs about 3 h after the middle of the light
period. It has been observed in whole and in anucleate
algae. The rhythm is readily lost in constant light of intensity equal to that given during the light period of the
normal light-dark cycle. However it has been shown that
the oscillation is not a direct consequence of the lightening regimen and, therefore, endogenous. The synthesis of
RNA is observed in these experiments,under light conditions, after short pulses of ^{3}H-uridine: it has been
shown to be associated with the chloroplasts (11).

The rhythm in photosynthesis

The rhythm in photosynthesis is the best documented of all rhythms in Acetabularia. It can be measured either by O_2 evolution or by CO_2 fixation (12-19) (fig.1). Both photosynthesis and photosynthetic capacity oscillate in parallel manner (19). The maximum occurs at the middle of the light period. The rhythm is typically circadian, easily kept in free-running conditions. The anucleate algae display the same rhythm as do whole ones, even 5 weeks after anucleation (15). Terborgh and Mc Leod (19) have shown that the natural period of the rhythm of photosynthesis in Acetabularia crenulata is approximately 25 h at 28°C.

The rhythm in chloroplast shape

The chloroplasts of Acetabularia mediterranea vary in shape with the time of the day (17) : they are more elongated in the middle of the light period and more spherical in the middle of the dark period. In order to evaluate the changes in chloroplasts shape, the ratios between the long and the short axis were calculated and their distribution curves were established. When the chloroplasts are more spherical, the distribution curve of the axis ratios lies between 1 and 4 ; when they are more elongated, the distribution curve is displaced and the axis ratios vary from 3 to 11.

The rhythm is endogenous and is maintained for two days at least when the algae are kept in constant light (17). Whole algae as well as anucleate fragments display the rhythm (18).

This rhythm is represented in fig.1. The measurements, in this particular experiment, have been made in the middle of the light period and in the middle of the dark period on comparable samples of algae simultaneously used for the determination of the rhythm in photosynthetic capacity, also represented in the fig. This experiment has been chosen as representative of concomitant variation of these two functions (18).

The rhythm in ATP content of the chloroplasts

The ATP content of the sedimentable fraction and of the supernatant has been studied in collaboration with E. Schram, using his new adaptation of the luciferin-luciferase method (21). It has been found (table 1) that the ATP content of the chloroplasts is significantly higher 5 hours before the middle of the light period than at the middle (content in ATP of the chloroplasts or on a chlorophyll weight basis). The ATP content of the supernatant varies in the opposite way. These oscillations are maintained in continuous light. The fact that the ATP content of the sedimentable fraction is higher in the morning than it is in the middle of the light cycle is very important since it points to the possible presence of another circadian rhythm that could use ATP to a higher extent than the increment resulting from the rhythm in photosynthesis. This point will be emphasized later on.

The rhythm in the polysaccharides of the sedimentable fraction

The insoluble carbohydrates of the chloroplasts were next investigated in collaboration with S. Bonotto: they are the main product of photosynthesis.

The chloroplasts separated either by centrifugation of whole homogenates or by density gradient on glycerol, then repeatedly washed with cold ethanol always react positively with the Selivanoff test (62). This reaction is fairly specific for fructosans i.e. it is about ten times more sensitive to fructose than it is to glucose.

Chromatography was performed on the ethanol washed sediments obtained from whole homogenates. After acid hydrolysis (HCl 0.5N), no fructose residues are detectable by the diphenylamine-aniline (in phosphoric acid) reaction. On the contrary, if a mild hydrolysis is conducted with sulfosalicylic acid, fructose residues only are detected on paper chromatograms with ethylacetate-pyridine-water. Control commercial soluble starch (Merck, Darmstadt) was hydrolysed under these conditions. Parallel chromatograms have shown that, in first approximation, there must be about 3 to 4

217

times more glucose residues than fructose residues after hydrolysis (HCl, 0.5 N) of the polymers. It has not been checked whether galactose residues are present : it has been shown by Shephard (22) that chloroplasts actively synthesize this sugar.

Obviously, much more work has to be done before the exact composition of the chloroplasts carbohydrates is known.

Experiments are undertaken in this Laboratory in order to follow the circadian variation of the polysaccharides by performing both the Selivanoff and the phenol tests on the sedimentable and the supernatant fractions of aliquot samples. The aim of these experiments is to determine whether only the fructosan fraction varies with the time of the day, or both the fructosans and the glucosans vary.

Using the Selivanoff test, it has been found that the sedimentable fraction contains polysaccharides varying with the time of the day (26). The maximum occurs at about 3 h after the middle of the light period, which is also the maximum in the photosynthetic rhythm (fig.2). The rhythm in polysaccharides is maintained in continuous light and, therefore, is typically endogenous. It is displayed by whole algae as well as by anucleate fragments.

Rhythm in the number of carbohydrate granules in the chloroplasts and in chloroplast division

Puiseux-Dao and Gilbert (23) have observed a daily variation in the number of chloroplasts containing 1, 2, 3 or more carbohydrate granules (fig.2). As Puiseux-Dao emphazised (24), the number of the chloroplastic granules is an easy reference to the number of the "plastidial units". The number of chloroplasts containing one granule decreases during the first hours of illumination ; at the same time the number of chloroplasts with 2 or more granules increases.

After a levelling off of the three curves, they all show a dramatic change: the number of chloroplasts containing one granule increases, while the converse is observed for the others. It is of interest to note that the maximum in polysaccharide content preceeds only slightly (one hour or less) the second inflexion point of the number of chloroplasts with one, two or several granules.

Puiseux-Dao considers that the period during which the proportion of one granule containing chloroplasts decreases at the expense of the chloroplasts with two or several granules corresponds to the replicative period of the plastidial unit. It could be suggested that the steady levels of the curves correspond to a G2 phase. Finally, the division of the plastidial units explains the increase in number of the chloroplasts with one granule and the decrease of those with more than one.

All the chloroplasts do not divide every day. Puiseux-Dao (25) has calculated that they can be assimilated to a population in exponential growth and dividing every 5 days. Division itself takes place at the tenth hour after the beginning of the light period.

The rhythm in division of the plastidial population is comparable to the rhythm of division of the cell population displayed by certain unicellular organisms.

Interdependence between rhythms

One should now examine whether or not certain rhythms could be merely dependent on others ; in other words, if there exist, in Acetabularia one or a number of oscillating functions.

Experiments performed in different light regimes and in the presence or the absence of inhibitors (18) have shown that photosynthesis and chloroplast shape are intimately related: the O_2 evolution and the shape of the organelle seem to be two manifestations of the same phenomenon.

Photosynthesis results in ATP synthesis. Whenever both the ATP content of the sediment and of the supernatant have been measured, it can be calculated that there is a general increase in total ATP content between the morning and the middle of the light period. However, ATP decreases in the sediment (fig 3). Therefore, another function or several other functions must oscillate in the chloroplasts and use ATP to a higher extent than the increment resulting from the rhythm in photosynthesis. One of these functions could be polysaccharide synthesis which would be oscillating independently.

Experiments of incorporation of ^{14}C-fructose into the

219

chloroplasts (in collaboration with S. Bonotto) show that
(1) the rate of incorporation varies with the time of the
day,
(2) this variation is endogenous, since it is observed in
algae kept in L:L as well as in algae maintained in L:D
and
(3) the incorporation rate is higher 3 h after the middle
of the light period than it is at the middle itself, suggesting that there could be an autonomous rhythm in polysaccharide synthesis.

If the existence of such an independent oscillation is
confirmed, it would be easier to understand the decrease
in chloroplastic ATP and the lag between the curves in
photosynthesis and in polysaccharide content.

As far as the circadian rhythm in RNA synthesis is concerned, its much more rapid damping in constant light, pro-
ves that it is independent of the other rhythms in particular, that it is not depending on the energy generated by
the photosynthesis.

Summarizing, we know 5 different main rhythms for
Acetabularia: the rhythm in photosynthesis and in chloroplast shape, intimately correlated, the rhythm in the polysaccharide content, as measured by the number of chloroplastic granules and in chloroplast's division, which are
apparently two aspects of the same rhythm, but probably not
entirely dependent to the above mentioned ones, and the
rhythm in RNA synthesis.

The variation in fructose incorporation is probably
responsible for the rhythm in the polysaccharide content.
The oscillation in the ATP content must depend on both the
rhythm in photosynthesis and at least one ∴other oscillation.

If these rhythms can be grouped, three oscillating systems became apparent, that could be geared by one basic
central mechanism. Alternatively, there could be three entraining basic mechanisms, each entraining one overt oscillation. In other words, Acetabularia displays a number of
overt rhythms entrained by one or several cellular "Biological Clocks".

Interpretation

The overt process
How can this scheme be interpreted in molecular terms?

A number of informations are available as for the synthetic processes. The rhythm in photosynthesis has been extensively studied. If no variation in the content in chlorophyll has ever been detected (unpublished experiments and 19), Hellebust et al (20) have recently shown that, in Acetabularia crenulata it must result of the concomitant variation in both light and dark reactions or in their coupling. No variation has been found in the in vitro activity of ribulose diphosphocarboxylase (as has been found to be the case in Gonyaulax, 58) nor in the activity of 8 other enzymes of the Calvin's cycle (20).

Since Acetabularia mediterranea displays rhythmicity, both in photosynthesis and in photosynthetic capacity, and since the rhythm in the shape of the chloroplasts is tightly linked to that in photosynthesis, it is conceivable that substructural variations parallel molecular distortions bringing about variations in the rate of energy transfer, or that variations in the electron transfer resulting in a mechano-chemical work modify the supramolecular organization.

It is not known if oscillating enzymes are operating in the synthesis of RNA. Similar rhythms have been observed in Phaseolus (29) and in Mammals (30).

In spite of the ignorance in which we are as to the proportion of fructosans and glucosans and, possibly, as to the presence of still other residues, it is conceivable that, in Acetabularia, one or several enzymes of the metabolism of carbohydrates are subjected to circadian variations, as it is known to be the case for starch (31) and glycogen (30, 32, 33, 34, 35). In the first instance, several enzymes have been found to oscillate in different systems : amylase (36-39), phosphorylase (40, 61), invertase (41), in the operation of the Embden-Mayerhof cycle (42). In the metabolism of glycogen also, several enzymes have been found to display a rhythmic activity (32, 43). An interesting correlation should be emphasized: most of the enzymes that have been found to oscillate with the time of the day are known to be allosteric proteins, phosphatases and phosphorylases for example.

As the overt processes seem to be supported by proteins and as they are, in the case of Acetabularia, located in the chloroplasts, two types of experiments have been performed. First, the effects of the inhibitors of the syn-

thesis of proteins have been investigated by Sweeney (13)
and by ourselves (44). It has been found after 24 or 48 h
that photosynthesis is severely decreased, which oblitera-
tes -but not completely supresses- the circadian rhythm :
the proteins indispensable for photosynthesis are no longer synthesized. A second approach was the study of the
effects of rifampicin. In vitro, rifampicin acts specifically on bacterial transcription, by binding to the RNA-
polymerase (45, 46, 47). Wehrli and coll. (48) have recently shown that the antibiotic not only interacts with the
enzyme but reduces bacterial growth, sometimes dramatically.

Using this antibiotic it has been hoped to inhibit a
rhythmic process in the chloroplast that would depend on
a chloroplastic m-RNA. As those of bacteria, chloroplastic
m-RNAs are supposed to be short-lived. The results of these
experiments are presented in table 2. The first figure is
the value of the photosynthetic capacity at 5 H before the
middle of the light period, the second figure is the photosynthetic capacity at the middle of the light period and
the third figure is the ratio of the first and the second:
it allows a comparison between the amplitude of the oscillations of the control and treated Acetabularia.

Rifampicin, at the concentration of 10 µg ml^{-1} during
three days or at the higher concentrations of 20 µg ml^{-1}
during 24 h had no effect on photosynthesis nor on rhythmicity. At the same time, it has been demonstrated that no
new chloroplastic RNA is synthesized (49). If chloroplastic
RNA contains short-lived m-RNAs coding for specific proteins, rhythmicity does not involve the synthesis of such
RNAs.

In conclusion, from the experiments with inhibitors of
translation and with the most specific inhibitor known of
transcription in chloroplasts, no positive result has been
obtained so far, concerning the rhythms manifested by the
chloroplasts of Acetabularia.

The basic mechanism of rhythmicity

Concerning the basic mechanism of rhythmicity interesting information has emerged from experiments with Acetabularia, owing to the fact that the cells withstand anucleation.

The nuclear control

The fact that anucleate fragments retain their rhythm
in photosynthesis is well known (12, 14, 15, 18). The same
holds true for the rhythm in chloroplast shape (18).

Actinomycin D has been tested on whole algae (18). This
specific inhibitor of transcription, at the concentration
of 0.27 μg ml^{-1} decreases the rhythm in photosynthetic
capacity-as that in chloroplast shape - within a few days,
and inhibits totally the rhythm in about 12 to 15 days ;
during that period, the RNA previously formed must have been
used up and no new molecules could be synthesized. Consequently, the system Biological Clock ⟶ Rhythmicity has
a definite turnover and depends on a RNA, probably a m-RNA.
The two types of experimental evidence (maintenance of
the rhythm during 6 weeks in anucleate Acetabularia and
during 2 weeks in actinomycin-treated whole algae) have led
to the hypotheses that (1) the rhythm depends on a specific
nuclear RNA and (2) the life-time of this specific RNA is
different in whole and in anucleate Acetabularia. These
hypotheses have been checked by two series of experiments:
1. Since actinomycin D inhibits the synthesis of RNA but
has no effect on preexisting RNAs, actinomycin D should
not affect the rhythm of anucleate algae. This, in fact is
the case : it has not been possible to detect any difference between control anucleate fragments and actinomycin-
treated anucleate fragments in the rhythms of both photosynthetic capacity and chloroplast shape (18).
2. The second evidence supporting these hypotheses results
from a grafting experiment (44). The nucleate rhizoid of
a strain endowed with rhythmicity (R$^+$) was grafted onto
the 2 to 3 cm long stalk of an alga of a strain without
rhythmicity (R$^-$). The converse experiment was also performed. There is only a small number of chloroplasts around
the nucleus of the graft as compared to the number of
chloroplasts in the 2.5 cm stalk. Before grafting, the R$^+$
strain displayed a rhythm equal to 2.4. After 19 to 21
days, the Acetabularia with a nucleus of an R$^+$ strain
displayed a photosynthetic rhythm of 2.1, which is
highly significant (17), whereas those with a

nucleus of the R⁻ strain had a photosynthetic rhythm of
1.45, which is not significant.

Confirmation of the nuclear control
and stimulation of rhythmicity

In another experimental series, the effects of RNase
have been examined. The direct effects of RNase are difficult to estimate, since photosynthesis itself decreases
sharply (the concentration used was 0.1 mg ml^{-1}). When algae were transferred to normal sea-water after treatment
with RNase, photosynthesis was resumed; but the anucleate
Acetabularia do not display any more rhythmicity. This is
a new evidence supporting the hypothesis that a nuclear
m-RNA is implicated in the control mechanism of circadian
rhythmicity. In contrast with this result, in whole algae,
the value of the rhythm is significantly higher than in
the controls, provided that the recovery period had been
sufficiently long (18).

This interesting result should be connected with the
following experiments: algae were sectioned in different
ways, only the apex, or half of the stalk, or leaving only
the nucleus. It has been found that fragmentation induces
a stimulation of the rhythm, the smaller the remaining
fragment, the greater the stimulation (50).

When the number of molecules of the specific m-RNA decreases, a compensatory mechanism operates, and a stimulation in the synthesis of the m-RNA takes place. This stimulation would result from a derepression of specific nuclear genes.

The experiments described above support the hypothesis
that a nuclear m-RNA controls the rhythms of the chloroplasts.

Absence of increase in rhythmicity in the apex

Brachet (60) demonstrated the existence of an apico-
basal gradient of nucleic acids; the nucleic acids are manufactured by the nucleus and are accumulated in the apex
of the alga. In order to test if such an apico-basal gradient could affect the rhythm, the following experiment
has been made: the algae were fragmented in such a way that

the apex is included in the fragment (anucleate apical
fragment) or not included (anucleate basal fragment).
No increase could be detected in the rhythm in photosynthetic capacity in the anucleate apical fragments as compared with the basal ones (50). The involved RNA must have
been very rapidly complexed either in the cytoplasm or in
the chloroplasts.

Phasing and setting the rhythm

Schweiger (51) very elegantly demonstrated that the
nucleus phases the photosynthesis rhythm in Acetabularia,
by three sets of experiments : first, algae had their
stalk and rhizoid submitted to illumination in opposite
phase, then transferred to constant light ; secondly,
stalks were transplanted to rhizoids originating from algae in opposite illumination phase, then transferred to
constant light and, thirdly, nuclei were implanted in anucleate stalks also in opposite phase and also transferred
thereafter in constant light. In all three cases the photosynthesis rhythm became in phase with that of the nucleus in about one week. It could be that a progressive
replacement of existing m-RNAs by new ones takes place,
their life-time being somewhat shorter than in our experiments, due to differences either in varietes or in culture conditions.
Light is the entraining agent "par excellence" and,
although the nucleus has a dramatic influence on the
phase, it has been observed, however (18), that anucleate
Acetabularia as well as whole algae are capable of reset-
ting the rhythm. This is compatible with the interpretation suggested here about the differential turn-over of
specific RNAs in whole algae and anucleate fragments.
Even setting of the rhythm is possible in anucleate fragments as demonstrated by Richter (14). The molecules responsible for rhythmicity, that have originated from the
nucleus, must have been stored in the cytoplasm and await
there the rhythm setting signal.

Summary

We can summarize all the results in a general scheme
(fig.4). If the classical DNA-RNA-proteins chain is

considered, the inhibitors of translation decrease the
value of the rhythmic response very rapidly, and do not
affect the period nor the phase. Newly synthesized proteins
could thus eventually embody one of the overt oscillators
(or part of it), which is coupled to the central basic
one. In this basic mechanism a nuclear RNA has a central
role. A feed-back mechanism regulates the synthesis of
RNA, in response to a loss. However, phasing and setting
the rhythm can occur in the absence of the nucleus.

General Interpretation

Do the results obtained with Acetabularia converge with
those obtained with other systems? Do they provide any clue
that would allow a general conclusion as for the operation
of rhythmicity? No mechanism has been unquestionably demonstrated. The prevalent ideas about circadian rhytmicity
will be summarized, the conclusions gained with Acetabularia
compared with those provided by other systems and, finally,
possible working hypotheses will be briefly discussed.

The intrinsic similarity of circadian rhythms in plants
and in animals is so striking, the unique character of the
phenomenon so conspicuous, that it is generally assumed
that a common mechanism underly all circadian rhythms.
Two main reciprocally exclusive tendencies are found in
the litterature. Brown and coworkers (52), on the basis of
the receptiveness of organisms to weak electromagnetic
fields (of the same order of magnitude that of the earth),
believe that circadian rhythms are not truly endogenous,
but mere responses to the interaction of geophysical factors, light and other environmental factors.

On the contrary, most authors believe that an intrinsic mechanism is responsible for the circadian rhythms and
assume that an internal "biological clock" regulates rhythmicity. As already mentioned, it might include two coupled
oscillators; Pittendrigh has contributed much evidence for
this duality (53). The chemical nature of the oscillators
as well as the mechanism generating the oscillations remain unknown. Hasting's experiments with Gonyaulax (54)
and Strumwasser's experiments with Aplysia (55), have
shown that, as in Acetabularia, RNA plays a central role.
Rhythms are sometimes suppressed by inhibitors of transcription, such as the rat liver tryptophan pyrrolase (56)
or by acting on translation, such as the zonation rhythm
in fungi (Jerebzoff, 57).

226

A comprehensive molecular model, was first proposed
by Ehret and Trucco in 1967 (28). They called it the
chronon concept. In this model, the temporal control results from the operation of two components : the chronon
or transcriptional component and the recycling component.
The transcription rate from a very long polycistronic
DNA segment is limited by a number of intercistronic
events that include diffusion of m-RNA from the nucleus to
the cytoplasm, translation of initiators for the following
transcriptional step and diffusion of initiator from the
cytoplasm to the nucleus. The recycling component compri-
ses translation, end product formation, polymer association, and accumulation of the initiator substance. The
model is thus a self-programming mechanism for the circadian escapement. This very stimulating model is in
agreement with a great number of observations, specially
about enzyme rhythms and in neuronal activity.

Acetabularia has proved unique from many points of
view. Whatever this model will be of general application
or not, it is not in agreement with the results obtained
with Acetabularia, since anucleate algae display rhythmicity as well as whole ones. It is unlikely that chloroplastic chronons operate in the absence of the nucleus
since no effect of rifampicin has been detected. Since
neither transcription nor translation seem to be implicated in the circadian escapement, search for a mechanism
should be directed towards more physical models. Experimental evidence suggest that RNA and porphyrins (59) are
components of the basic mechanism in Acetabularia.

In the case of this alga, it seems likely that the
molecules supporting the overt manifestations of the
various rhythms are proteic in nature and, possibly, allosteric; the coupling between the central mechanism and
the overt processes could be visualized, if this were the
case, as the release or the binding of effectors or re-
pressors, onto the proteins and directed in some way by
the basic mechanism.

It should be mentioned that the possible relevance
of the oscillations of the type observed by Chance
(64, 65) in NADH in yeast and sustained by a feed-back
mechanism should be investigated, although the two
types of rhythms seem to be in contrast : (1) the

circadian rhythms of which the period (of about 24 h) is not dependent on the concentration of enzymes or metabolites and (2) the short oscillations in yeast of which the period can be manipulated by enzyme or certain metabolite concentrations. Possibly, all rhythms in fungi are related to the latter: their period, though much longer than in Chance's system is also dependent on the concentration of the medium (57, 66). The two types of rhythm also manifest temperature sensitivity.

Few evidence has been obtained so far as to the nature of the molecules embodying the rhythms. RNA has a role of major importance in the elaborate device of regulation of activity, rhytmicity. Many new experiments will be necessary in order to understand its molecular operation.

Acknowledgements

The author expresses her thanks to Mr L. Lateur for culturing the Acetabularia, and to Miss M. Hayet for performing the measurements of ATP.

References

1. Brachet J. Bull. Acad. Roy. Belg. 49 : 862, 1963.
2. Clauss H. Protoplasma 65 : 49, 1968.
3. Terborgh J. and Thimann K. Planta 63 : 83, 1964
4. Terborgh J. Nature 207 : 1360, 1965.
5. Bünning E. Cold Spring Harbor Symposia Quant. Biol. 25 : 248, 1960.
6. Hammer K.C. and Takimoto A. Amer. Naturalist 98 : 295, 1964.
7. Ketellapper H.J. and Chang D.M. Planta 63 : 344, 1964.
8. Miller J.H. Amer. Journ. Bot. 47 : 532, 1969.
9. Halberg F. The Cellular Aspects of Biorhythms (H. von Mayersbach ed.) p. 20, Springer 1967.
10. Vanden Driessche T. and Bonotto S. Biochim. Biophys. Acta 179 : 58, 1969.

11. Bonotto S. Thèse de doctorat, Université Libre de Bruxelles, Fac. des Sciences, 1969.
12. Sweeney B.M. and Haxo F.T. Science 134 : 1361, 1961.
13. Sweeney B.M., Tuffli C.F. Jr. and Rubin R.H. J. Gen. Physiol. 50 : 647, 1967.
14. Richter G. Z.Naturforsch. 18b : 1085, 1963.
15. Schweiger E., Walraff, H.G. and Schweiger, H.G. Z. Naturforsch. 196 : 499, 1964.
16. Schweiger H.G. and Schweiger E. Proc. Feldafing Summer School (J. Aschoff ed.): p.195 North Holland Publ. Co. 1965.
17. Vanden Driessche T. Exptl. Cell. Res. 42 : 18, 1966.
18. Vanden Driessche T. Biochim. Biophys. Acta 126 : 456, 1966.
19. Terborgh J. and Mc Leod G.C. Biol. Bull. 133 : 659, 1967.
20. Hellebust J.A. Terborgh J. and Mc Leod G.C. Biol.Bull. 133 : 670, 1967.
21. Schram E. Proc. Symposium Liquid Scintillation Counting, Boston 1969. In press.
22. Shephard D.C., Levin W.B. and Bidwell R.G.S. Biochem. Biophys. Res. Comm. 32 : 413, 1968.
23. Puiseux-Dao, S.J. et Gilbert A.M. C.R. Acad. Sc. Paris, D, 265 : 870, 1967.
24. Puiseux-Dao S.J., 6th Internat. Congress Electron Microscopy, Kyoto : 377, 1966.
25. Puiseux-Dao S.J. C.R. Acad. Sc. Paris, D, 266 : 1382, 1968.
26. Vanden Driessche T.and Bonotto S. Arch.Internat. Physiol. Biochim. 76 : 205, 1968.
27. Bruce V.G. Proc. Feldafing Summer School (J. Aschoff ed.): p.125 North Holland Publ. Co. 1965.
28. Ehret C.F. and Trucco E. J. Theoret. Biol. 15 : 240, 1967.
29. Rückbeil A. Z. Botanik 49 : 1, 1961.
30. Halberg F., Halberg E., Barnum C.P. and Bittner J.J. Photoperiodism and related phenomena in plants and in animals. Amer. Ass. Adv. Sc. p.803 2e ed. 1961.
31. Bünning E. Die Physiologische Uhr, Springer 1963.
32. Mayersbach von H. Cellular aspects of Biorhythms : 87, Springer 1966.
33. Agren G. Biochem. Z. 281 : 367, 1935.
34. Leske R. Excerpta medica 70 : 103, 1963.

35. Sollberger A. Annals N.Y. Acad. Sc. 117 : 519, 1964
36. Bünning E. Z. Botanik 37 : 433, 1942.
37. Ehrenberg M. Planta 38 : 244, 1950.
38. Ehrenberg M. Planta 43 : 528, 1964.
39. Venter J., Z. Botanik 44 : 59, 1956.
40. Viswanathan P.N., Srivastava L.M. and Krishmann P.S. Plant Physiol. 37 : 283, 1962.
41. Slack C.R. Austr. J. Biol. Sci. 18 : 781, 1965.
42. Sanwal G.G. and Krishman P.S. Nature 188 : 664, 1960.
43. Watanabe M., Potter V.R. and Pitot H.C. J. Nutrition 95 : 207, 1968.
44. Vanden Driessche T. Nach. Akad. Wissen. Göttingen 10 : 108, 1967.
45. Hartmann G., Honikel K.O., Knüsel F. and Nüesch J. Biochim. Biophys. Acta 145 : 843, 1967.
46. Wehrli W., Knüsel F., Schmid K. and Staehelin M. Proc. Nat. Acad. Sci. U.S. 61 : 667, 1968.
47. Di Mauro E., Snyder L., Marino P., Lamberti A., Coppo A. and Tocchini-Valentini G.P. Nature 222 : 533, 1968.
48. Wehrli W., Knüsel F. and Staehelin M. Biochem. Biophys. Res. Comm. 32 : 284, 1968.
49. Bonotto S., Janowski M., Vanden Driessche T. and Brachet J. Arch. Internat. Physiol. Biochim. 76 : 919, 1968.
50. Vanden Driessche T. Sci. Prog. Oxf. 55 : 293, 1967.
51. Schweiger H.G. Science 146 : 658, 1964.
52. Brown F.A. Jr. Canad. J. Bot. 47 : 287, 1969.
53. Pittendrigh C.S., Proc. Feldafing Summer School (J. Aschoff ed) : p.277. North Holland Publ. Co. 1965.
54. Hastings J.W. & Keynan A. Proc. Feldafing Summer School (J. Aschoff ed) : p.167. North Holland Publ. Co. 1965.
55. Strumwasser F. Proc. Feldafing Summer School (J. Aschoff ed.) p.443. North Holland Publ. Co. 1965.
56. Rensing L. Nature 219 : 619, 1968.
57. Jerebzoff S. Proc. Feldafing Summer School (J. Aschoff ed.) p.183. North Holland Publ. Co. 1965.
58. Sweeney B.M. Proc. Feldafing Summer School (J. Aschoff ed.) : p.190. North Holland Publ. Co. 1965.
59. Hastings J.W. and Sweeney B.M. J. Gen. Physiol. 43 : 697, 1960.
60. Brachet J. Progr. Biophys. Molec. Biol. 15 : 97, 1965.
61. Richter G. and Pirson A. Flora 144 : 562, 1957.
62. Yaphé W. and Arsenault G.P. Anal. Biochem. 13 : 143, 1965.

63. Dubois M., Gilles K.A., Hamilton J.K., Rebers P.A. and Smith F. Anal. Chem. 28 : 350, 1956.
64. Chance B., Schoener B. and Elsaesser S. J. Biol.Chem. 240:3170, 1965.
65. Chance B., Pye K. and Higgins J. IEEE Spectrum 4 : 76, 1967.
66. Nguyen Van H. Thèse de la Fac. Sc.Orsay, Université de Paris, sé. A, n° 291, 1967.

Table 1

ATP content of Acetabularia at the beginning
and at the middle of the light period

Exper.	ATP content of the chloroplasts (pM of ATP per 100 μg of chlorophyll) and standard deviation between brackets			ATP content of the supernatant (pM per 20 algae)		
	time t.1	time t.2	ratio 2/1	time t.1	time t.2	ratio 2/1
I	6.30 (1.90)	3.55 (1.23)	1.8			
II	7.26 (1.33)	4.41 (-)	1.6			
III	4.37 (-)	2.88 (-)	1.5	600	898	0.7
IV	4.49 (0.36)	2.99 (0.69)	1.5	724	860	0.8

The mean values were obtained from 3 samples of 20 algae, except in the cases where no standard deviation has been calculated, for which 2 samples were available.
Lightning regime, L:D = 12:12
Light period, from 9 to 18
Time of the measurements : t.1,9.30 in experiment 1,9.00 in the other experiments
t.2, between 14.30 and 15,30

Table 2

The effect of rifampicin on the photosynthetic capacity of <u>Acetabularia</u>

Exper.	Controls	1 µg.ml^{-1}, 24 h	10 µg.ml^{-1}, 24 h	10 µg.ml^{-1}, 3 d	20 µg.ml^{-1}, 24 h
I	11.78	13.27	12.62		
	18.74	20.26	20.01		
	1.6	1.5	1.6		
II	24.72		29.95		
	33.58		31.78		
	1.4		1.1		
V	19.28	17.79	20.48		17.47
	28.35	31.10	26.62		26.95
	1.5	1.7	1.3		1.5
VI	15.46		14.93		
	18.81		19.09		
	1.2		1.3		
VII	14.94			11.32	
	17.70			17.53	
	1.2			1.55	

Each 3 superposed values are respectively : the mean photosynthesis rate (µl of O_2 evol-ved by 25 algae in 30 min.) at 5 h before the middle of the light period, at the middle of the light period and the ratio of these two rates.

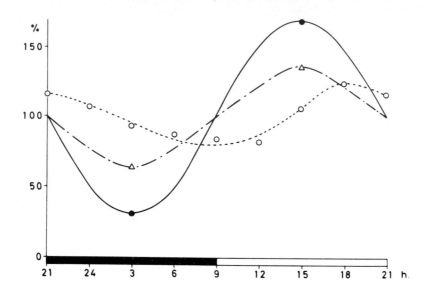

Fig.1. Time-map of <u>Acetabularia</u> 1.

Rhythm in photosynthetic capacity: solid line with solid circles.
Rhythm in chloroplast shape: broken line with open triangles.
Rhythm in RNA synthesis: dotted line and open circles.
The relative values of the two first rhythms have been calculated from aliquot samples in a representative experiment reported in (17).
The relative values of the RNA synthesis are calculated from a typical experiment reported in (10).

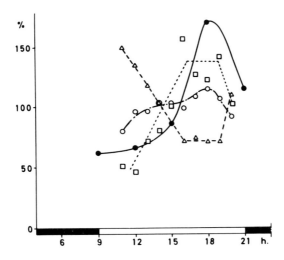

Fig.2. Time-map of <u>Acetabularia</u> 2.

Rhythm in the polysaccharide content of the chloroplasts:
solid line with solid circles.
Rhythm in the number of chloroplastic granules: chloroplasts with one granule, broken line with open triangles –
chloroplasts with two granules, broken line with open
circles – chloroplasts with three or several granules,
dotted line with open squares.
The relative values of the rhythm in polysaccharide content is a representative experiment.
The curves of the relative values concerning the number of
granules per chloroplast are derived from the work of
Puiseux-Dao and Gilbert (23) where the original values are
the means of three experimental series.

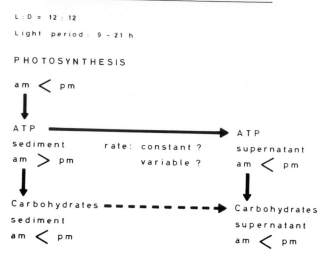

Fig.3. Photosynthesis, ATP content and polysaccharide con-
    tent of the chloroplasts and of the cytoplasm in
Acetabularia (mitochondrial ATP has not been taken into
account, respiration in Acetabularia, in the experimental
conditions used, being small as compared with photosynthesis).

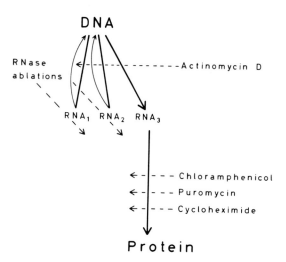

Fig.4. Regulation of temporal activity in Acetabularia.
    Tentative scheme.

AFTERNOON SESSION

Chairman: Jean-René Maisin

AMINO ACIDS INCORPORATION BY CHLOROPLASTS ISOLATED FROM ANUCLEATE ACETABULARIA[x]

André Goffeau

EURATOM, Biology, Brussels, Belgium

and

Laboratoire de Morphologie Animale,
Université Libre de Bruxelles,
Brussels, Belgium.

Abstract

Chloroplasts isolated from anucleate fragments of the giant unicellular alga Acetabularia mediterranea actively incorporate radioactive amino acids. A systematic study of the conditions necessary for obtaining active isolated chloroplasts is reported. Microbiological and electron microscopy controls, as well as the absence of inhibition by streptomycin and the requirements of magnesium ions and an amino acid mixture, permit to reject the hypothesis of an artefact due to bacterial contamination of the chloroplasts suspension.

The effectiveness of actinomycin D, puromycin and chloramphenicol, specific inhibitors of certain stages in protein synthesis prompts the conclusion that the chloroplast protein synthesis system requires the participation of DNA, transfer RNA and ribosomes. These nucleic acids are most probably localised in the chloroplasts.

The incorporation of amino acids by isolated chloroplasts is inhibited by chloramphenicol and tetracycline, inhibitors of bacterial ribosomal systems. On the other hand, cycloheximide, a specific inhibitor of cytoplasmic ribosomal system in higher organisms, has no effect.

x Publication n° 480 of EURATOM, Biology, Brussels

239

Isolated <u>Acetabularia</u> chloroplasts incorporate amino acids not only in their structural protein fraction but also in other membrane-bound and soluble proteins. From comparison of the specific radioactivities it is concluded that the chloroplast DNA codes not only for proteins of the chloroplast structural protein fraction but also for other water-insoluble proteins as well as water-soluble proteins.

Our results on isolated <u>Acetabularia</u> chloroplasts are different from those obtained with isolated mitochondria, where the amino acids are incorporated into the insoluble protein fraction only. Our results suggest that chloroplast DNA codes for more proteins than mitochondrial DNA. As a result, the growth of the chloroplasts would be less dependent on the nucleus than that of the mitochondria.

Introduction

<u>Acetabularia</u> is a convenient living material in several different respects. Not only it can furnish viable anucleate fragments but its chloroplasts are remarquably resistant to mechanical and chemical damage. This property allows one to obtain well preserved isolated chloroplasts with an almost total recovery (1, 2). Electron micrographs of chloroplasts isolated from anucleate fragments of <u>Acetabularia mediterranea</u> show at least three states or types of chloroplast (fig. 1). The type 1 chloroplasts are loose and do not reveal any membranous structure. In type 2, the lamellae and the outer membrane are quite distinct. The type 3 chloroplasts are very dense and contracted. This heterogenity is similar to what is observed with isolated mitochondria (3). The presence of some mitochondria and of cytoplasmic islands is also noticeable. The outer membrane is unusually stable in <u>Acetabularia</u> chloroplasts; the majority of isolated chloroplasts still possess their outer membrane. <u>Acetabularia</u> chloroplasts are not disrupted unlike most higher plant species, in hypotonic conditions. Moreover, 1 % Triton 100 does not fragment the <u>Acetabularia</u> chloroplasts which still sediment out in 5 min at 1,000 g although the chlorophylls are completely solubilized. This unusual behaviour suggests

240

that the outer chloroplastic membrane of Acetabularia has
a different chemical composition than the outer membrane
of chloroplasts of higher plants.

Isolated Acetabularia chloroplasts incorporate a
mixture of labelled amino acids very rapidly into their
proteins[x]. The chloroplasts (isolated from 20 algae)
incorporate amino acids 20 times faster than the supernatant of the 1000 g centrifugation which contains all the
cytoplasmic elements lighter than the chloroplasts. The
rate of incorporation of radioactive amino acids by chloroplasts isolated from anucleate fragments is constant for
at least the first 30 min and decreases somewhat thereafter (fig. 2A). The incorporation is related to the chlorophyll concentration up to 25 µg chlorophyll per ml of
reaction mixture (fig. 2B).

Optimal experimental conditions

Several factors are important in order to obtain
high amino acids incorporation rates into proteins by
isolated Acetabularia chloroplasts.

The pH during homogenizing is essential : amino
acid incorporation in chloroplasts isolated from homogenates grinded at pH 5.9 is only one half as efficient as
that of chloroplasts prepared at pH 6.4. This is probably
due to the acidity (pH 2-3) of the central vacuole of
Acetabularia (4).

The presence of about 10 mM of magnesium in the
reaction mixture is a necessary requirement for the incorporation (Table I).

We also noticed that no incorporation could be observed when single radioactive amino acids (leucine,
arginine or valine) were used instead of a mixture of 15
different amino acids. These observations suggest that
the internal pool of magnesium and soluble amino acids
either are limited in vivo or are washed out during the
isolation of the chloroplasts.

---

[x] The methods are described in more detail in references
1 and 2.

When isolated chloroplasts are disrupted by a brief
sonication prior to the incubation, the amino acid incorporation is reduced to 10 % of its original rate (fig. 3).
This inactivation is not due to the dilution of the chloroplast ATP or GTP since the addition of these nucleotides
does not stimulate the activity of the fragmented chloroplasts. Moreover, a simple preincubation at 25°C for 30
min of the reaction mixture in the absence of amino acids
reduces the activity of isolated chloroplasts to only 38 %
of that of control chloroplasts kept at 0°C. This treatment probably induces changes of the chloroplastic structure (e.g. by swelling). These results suggest that the
protein synthesis system is closely integrated in the
chloroplast structure and that its activity is closely
dependent on the integrity of this structure.

Contamination of the chloroplast fraction

In higher plants it is difficult to distinguish the
incorporation due to chloroplasts from that due to contaminating bacteria, intact cells, nuclei, mitochondria,
endoplasmic reticulum and other structures. In Acetabularia
the problem of contamination is greatly simplified. By
filtering the crude extract on a nylon bolting silk of
15 µ pore size, one completely excludes contamination by
whole cells and cells walls. Since only a nucleate algae
are used, the chloroplastic fraction is free of any nuclear
contamination. Electron micrographs of the chloroplast
pellet show the presence of a few mitochondria and fragments of the endoplasmic reticulum. But these contamina-
tions cannot contribute much to the observed amino acid
incorporation since the activity of the 1,000 - 10,000 g
pellet, which is enriched in mitochondria is considerably
lower than the chloroplastic pellet. Participation of cytoplasmic ribosomes or microsomes seems to be excluded since
the incorporation of amino acid by the chloroplastic fraction is completely insensitive to ribonuclease at concentrations up to 200 µg/ml (fig. 4).

The possible contamination by bacteria is a more
serious problem. Warning of the presence of bacteria in
chloroplast fractions has been given by App and Jagendorf
(5). However, we believe that in our working conditions
the bacterial contamination is negligible. Less than 20

bacteria capable of forming colonies on several agar mediums have been detected per reaction mixture. Furthermore, the rate of amino acids incorporation by isolated chloroplasts is only slightly sensitive to streptomycin which is known to inhibit bacterial protein synthesis. In order to eliminate the possible presence of streptomycin resistant bacteria in the chloroplast suspension, it has been checked that streptomycin strongly inhibits (70 %) the amino acid incorporation into bacteria obtained from non sterile Acetabularia. Moreover, the absolute requirements of magnesium and of a mixture of amino acids are not expected for bacterial amino acid incorporation. Finally, the inhibition of amino acids incorporation by a 30 minutes aging of the isolated chloroplasts, and the lack of effect of further washings of the chloroplasts, which should diminish some of the possible bacterial contaminants, also disfavour the hypothesis of a significant bacterial contamination. These evidences are reinforced by the examination of electron micrographs of the chloroplastic pellet, where no bacteria could be detected.

Effects of inhibitors

The action of the different inhibitors permits some insight of the mechanisms involved in the amino acids incorporation by isolated Acetabularia chloroplasts. This amino acids incorporation is sensitive to actinomycin D, puromycin, chloramphenicol and tetracycline. On the other hand, it is insensitive to penicillin, streptomycin and cycloheximide (fig. 5).

Since amino acid incorporation is carried out by chloroplasts obtained from algae anucleated as long as thirty days earlier, this incorporation must be not directly dependent on nuclear DNA. However, this fact does not necessarily imply that the chloroplastic protein synthesis is under the control of the chloroplastic DNA. A stable messenger RNA coded by the nucleus could be still in operation in the anucleate algae. This stable nuclear messenger RNA could be sticking on the surface of the chloroplasts.

The use of actinomycin D permits one to rule out this possibility. It is generally accepted that actinomycin D acts at the DNA level (6). Since, actinomycin D inhibits the incorporation of amino acids by chloroplasts isolated from Acetabularia, it seems that, at least after this time, the in vitro synthesis of chloroplastic proteins is dependent on chloroplastic DNA. However, since rather high concentrations of actinomycin D are necessary to produce inhibition, it is possible that the chloroplastic DNA has certain chemical or physical characteristics different from those of chromosomal DNA.

Puromycin inhibits protein synthesis in bacteria by competing with the amino-acyl-transfer RNA (AAsRNA) complex to which it has a structural similarity. Puromycin is thus able to mimic an incoming molecule of AAsRNA and forms a derivative of the polypeptide which will no longer be bound the ribosome (7). The sensitivity of the amino acid incorporation by isolated chloroplasts suggests that sRNA are also involved in the chloroplastic protein synthesized system.

The action of chloramphenicol in bacterial systems is not completely understood, but it interferes at the ribosomal level. It binds specifically to the 50 S subunit of the ribosomes and seems to disturb the attachment of the messenger RNA (8). Since the amino acid incorporation by isolated chloroplasts is chloramphenicol sensitive, this result indicates that ribosomes participate in the chloroplastic system. The fact that higher plants and animal cytoplasmic systems are not sensitive to chloramphenicol suggests that the chloroplastic synthesizing system is of the bacterial type. The chloroplastic protein synthesizing system seems thus to be somewhat distinct from the cytoplasmic system of green cells. Indeed, chloroplasts contain 70 S type ribosomes while the cytoplasm contains 80 S type ribosomes (9). The apparent specific inhibition by chloramphenicol of the chloroplastic and mitochondrial protein synthesis systems, has been widely used, recently, to differentiate these systems from the cytoplasmic protein synthesis (10, 11, 12).

Linnane and Stewart (13) have presented some evidences obtained in vivo that suggest that several antibiotics, among them tetracycline, have a specific action similar to that of chloramphenicol on the chloroplastic protein synthesizing system. Our results obtained in vitro support this concept. Moreover Clark - Walker and Linnane (14) have reported that in yeast the mitochondrial protein synthesis is unaffected by cycloheximide which seems to be a specific inhibitor of the cytoplasmic ribosomal system. Our results show that, in vitro, the chloroplastic protein synthesis system is unaffected by concentrations of cycloheximide up to 100 µg/ml, although in vivo the same concentration of cycloheximide kills the anucleate algae in a few days (15). Our in vitro results support thus the concept that in the chloroplastic protein synthesis systhem, as well in mitochondria, cycloheximide is not inhibitory and is a specific inhibitor of the cytoplasmic ribosomal system. However, when the inhibitors are incubated for two days with nucleate or anucleate Acetabularia fragments, neither cycloheximide nor chloramphenicol or tetracycline seem to be the specific inhibitors for the amino acids incorporation into the chloroplastic fraction (15). The reasons for this apparent discrepancy of the in vivo and in vitro results are not clear.

In conclusion, from the results obtained by the use of inhibitors, one may reasonably conclude that in isolated chloroplasts, the synthesis of chloroplastic protein is directed by chloroplastic DNA and that it is mediated by messenger, ribosomal and transfer RNAs. These different species of RNA are located within the chloroplasts and at least one of them, the ribosomal RNA, may manifests some differences from the cytoplasmic ribosomal RNA. However, the whole chloroplastic protein synthesizing system appears to be very similar to the bacterial system.

Fractionation of labelled proteins

It is now clear that the synthesis of mitochondrial proteins is under the combined control of both nucleic genes and mitochondrial DNA (see review 16). However it seems that in vitro, only the insoluble fraction (17, 18), in particular the so-called mitochondrial structural protein is synthesized (18, 19, 20, 21). The situation seems different for the Acetabularia chloroplasts where both soluble and membrane bound proteins are labelled in vitro (Table II). Since the algae were anucleated several days before the experiment, the presence of any nuclear DNA is excluded in our chloroplasts suspension. Moreover, since the in vitro incorporation of amino acids by isolated chloroplasts is RNAse insensitive the possibility that an active nuclear messenger RNA is sticking to the outside of the chloroplast surface is also disfavoured. The fact that the incorporation by isolated chloroplasts is independent of the time of enucleation (Table III) does also exclude the participation of a messenger RNA of nuclear origin in our in vitro system; in this case one would expect a decay of activity after long periods of enucleation. This of course does not necessarily mean that the in vivo genesis and replication of chloroplasts does not require the participation of cytoplasmic ribosomes and RNA. One may however reasonably assume that after isolation, chloroplasts manifest only their own independent protein synthesis. In other words, all of the proteins which are labelled in our in vitro system are under the control of chloroplastic DNA and are synthesized inside the chloroplasts. Since both soluble and membrane-bound proteins are labelled in vitro (Table II), we therefore conclude that the synthesis of both soluble and membrane-bound proteins is under chloroplastic protein synthesis system control. The table IV shows that the specific activity of amino acid incorporation into the membranous fraction is higher than in the soluble fraction. It appears thus that the membrane-bound proteins are the most actively synthesized in vitro.

Significant radioactivity has been found in every fraction that was obtained during the purification of the chloroplastic structural protein fraction according to Criddle's procedure (22). Table V shows that this "structural protein fraction" prepared from isolated Acetabularia chloroplasts has an amino acid composition rather similar to the chloroplast lamellar protein composition of other species (23, 24). One may conclude that at least one of the components of the chloroplastic structural protein fraction is among the membranous proteins which are coded by the chloroplastic DNA and synthesized within the chloroplasts. The specific radioactivity of the structural protein is lower than that of the total membranous fraction. This suggests that some membrane components not present in the structural protein fraction are more actively synthesized in vitro than the ones of the structural protein fraction.

As already pointed out, our results on isolated Acetabularia chloroplasts are different from those obtained by other authors with isolated mitochondria, where the amino acids seem to be incorporated into the insoluble protein fraction only. Since chloroplast DNA is 30 times larger than mitochondrial DNA (see review 25), it seems likely that, as our results suggest, chloroplast DNA codes for more proteins than mitochondrial DNA. As a result, the growth of the chloroplasts would be less dependent on the nucleus than that of the mitochondria.

However, another possibility has to be taken into consideration. The structural protein can form complexes having very different solubilities (22); it is conceivable that the labelled soluble and insoluble fractions correspond to different complexes of the structural protein, some of which could have been artificially created during purification. Further studies are necessary to test this hypothesis.

References

1. A. Goffeau and J. Brachet, Bioch. Bioph.Acta, 95, 302 (1965).
2. A. Goffeau, Bioch. Bioph. Acta 174, 340 (1969).
3. P. Wlodamer, D.F. Parsons, G.R. Williams and L. Wojtezak, Bioch. Bioph. Acta 128, 34 (1966).
4. J. Crawley, Exptl. Cell. Res. 32, 368 (1963).
5. A.A. App and A.T. Jagendorf, Bioch. Bioph. Acta 76, 286 (1963).
6. E. Reich and I.H. Goldberg, in Progress in Nucleic Acid Research and Molecular Biology, 3, 183 (1964) Academic Press.
7. D. Nathans, Proc. Natl. Ac. Sci. U.S., 51, 585 (1964).
8. D. Vazquez, Nature, 203, 257 (1964).
9. M.L. Peterman, in the Physical and Chemical Properties of Ribosomes, 19 (1964) Elsevier.
10. G. Clark-Walker and A. Linnane, J. Cell Biol. 34, 1 (1967).
11. M. Huang, D. Biggs, G. Clark-Walker and A. Linnane, Bioch. Bioph. Acta, 114, 434 (1966).
12. R. Smillie, D. Grahan, M. Duryer, A. Grieve and N. Tobin, Bicch. Bioph. Res. Comm., 28, 604 (1967).
13. A. Linnane and P.R. Stewart, Bioch. Bioph. Res. Comm., 27, 511 (1967).

14. G. Clark-Walker and A. Linnane, Bioch. Bioph. Res. Comm., 25, 535 (1967).
15. S. Bonotto, A. Goffeau, M. Janowski, T. Vanden Driessche and J. Brachet, Bioch. Bioph. Acta, 174, 704 (1969).
16. A. Goffeau, Année Biologique, 8, 10 (1969).
17. D.E. Truman, Biochem. J., 91, 59 (1964).
18. D.B. Roodyn, Biochem. J., 85, 177 (1962).
19. B. Kadenbach, Bioch. Bioph. Acta, 134, 430 (1967).
20. D. Haldar, K. Reeman and T.S. Work, Nature, 211, 9 (1966).
21. W. Neupert, D. Brdiczka and T. Bucher, Bioch. Bioph. Res. Comm., 27, 488 (1967).
22. R.S. Criddle, in Biochemistry of Chloroplasts, 203 (1966) Ed. by T. Goodwin, Ac. Press.
23. P. Weber, Z. Naturf., 18 b, 1105 (1963).
24. A. Lockshin and R.H. Burris, Proc. Natl. Ac. Sc. U.S., 56, 1564 (1966).
25. S. Granick and A. Gibor, in Progress in Nucleic Acid Research and Molecular Biology, 6, 143 (1967).

TABLE I

Influence of $MgCl_2$ in the reaction mixture on the incorporation of amino acids by chloroplasts isolated from anucleate fragments of Acetabularia

µmoles $MgCl_2$ per ml	Incorporation of amino acids (counts/min per h and per mg chlorophyll)
0	64 300
0.2	10 000
2	1 400
20	252 000
200	267 000

TABLE II

Distribution of radioactivity between soluble
and particulate proteins

Fractions	cpm in proteins	% of total cpm	
1,000 g supernatant	164.775	100	%
125,000 g pellet (particulate proteins)	97.844	60	%
125,000 g supernatant (soluble proteins)	55.750	34	%
1st wash of the 125,000 g pellet	3.217	2	%
2nd wash of the 125,000 g pellet	453	0,3	%
		recovery 96	%

TABLE III

Effect of anucleation on the relative incorporation into particulate proteins

Time of anucleation	10^3 cpm/hour and mg chl.	radioactivity into particulate proteins
1 day	816	60
11 days	692	51
18 days	801	58
25 days	811	57

TABLE IV

Specific radioactivities of protein fractions of isolated
<u>Acetabularia</u> chloroplasts incubated with labelled amino
acid[x]

Fraction	cpm incorporated/mg of proteins
Whole chloroplasts	8 000
Water soluble proteins	2 100
Water insoluble proteins (membrane fraction)	39 000
Membrane fraction soluble in 0,3 % SDS and 3 % urea	6 700
Membrane fraction insoluble in 0,3 % SDS and 3 % urea	83 000
Structural protein fraction	4 100

[x] The chloroplastic structural protein fraction was purified according to Criddle's procedure (22).

TABLE V

Amino acid composition of lamellar proteins preparations from Acetabularia and higher plants species

	Acetabularia Structural protein	Anthirrhinum (ref.23) Lamellar particle	Corn (ref.24) Lamellar protein	Spinach (ref.22) Structural protein
Lysine	4,9	3,8	4,7	8,2
Histidine	1,5	1,1	1,2	2,1
Arginine	3,9	3,8	4,5	1,0
Aspartic acid	9,3	8,9	7,7	14,0
Threonine	5,6	4,9	5,4	3,7
Serine	6,0	5,7	5,7	5,5
Glutamic acid	11,0	9,9	7,9	13,1
Proline	5,3	6,1	5,1	5,1
Glycine	11,0	11,2	9,3	9,2
Alanine	11,0	9,8	8,4	10,4
Valine	7,4	8,3	5,2	7,4
Methionine	traces	1,7	1,2	0,2
Isoleucine	5,8	4,5	4,4	6,6
Leucine	10,1	11,0	9,4	11,4
Tyrosine	1,6	1,8	2,7	0,7
Phenylalanine	5,8	6,2	5,1	0,2
Cysteic acid	–	–	0,5	1,3
Tryptophane	–	1,5	1,8	–

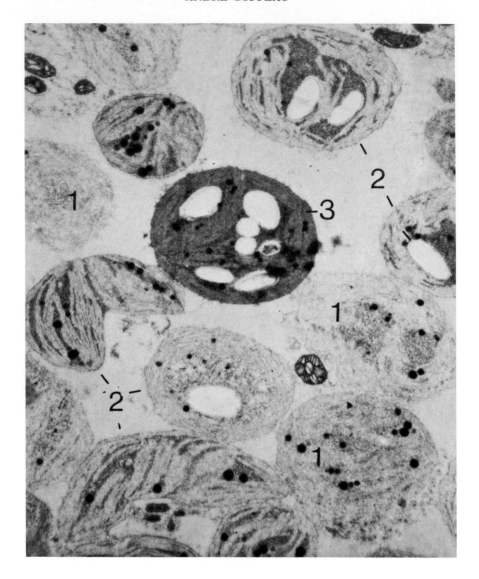

Fig. 1.   Electron micrograph of a pellet of washed unbroken Acetabularia chloroplasts.
The chloroplasts were isolated as usual, fixed by glutaraldehyde 3 % for 2 hours and osmium tetroxide 1 % for 1 hour, embeded in araldite, constrasted by uranyl acetate lead citrate. Magnification : 11.500'x.

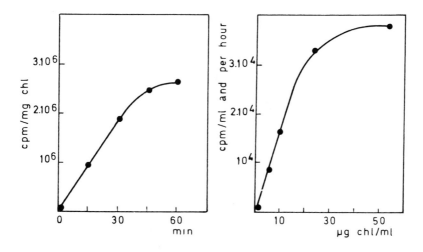

Fig. 2A. Time course of the incorporation of amino acids by chloroplasts isolated from anucleate fragments of Acetabularia. Algae anucleated for 5 days.
          2B. Incorporation of amino acids by chloroplasts isolated from anucleate fragments of Acetabularia versus chlorophyll concentration. Algae anucleated for 2 days.

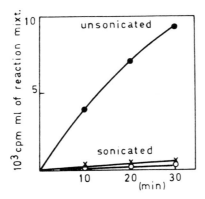

Fig. 3.   Inactivation of chloroplasts by sonication. Sonicated chloroplasts were treated for 30 seconds with a MSE sonifier at 5°C and centrifuged at 1,000 g for 5 minutes. 0.5 ml of the 1,000 g supernatant containing 20 μg of chlorophyll was used.

253

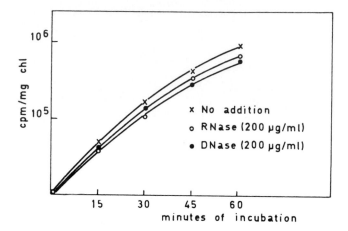

Fig. 4. Lack of inhibition by ribonuclease and deoxyribonuclease of the incorporation of amino acids by chloroplasts isolated from anucleate fragments of <u>Acetabularia</u>. Algae anucleated for 12 days. The reactions mixture contained 47 µg chlorophyll.

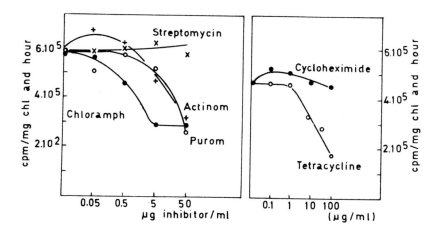

Fig. 5. Inhibition by protein synthesis inhibitors of the amino acids incorporation by chloroplasts isolated from anucleate fragments of <u>Acetabularia</u>.

EFFECTS OF GAMMA- RADIATION
ON ACETABULARIA MEDITERRANEA

Silvano Bonotto and René Kirchmann

Département de Radiobiologie
Centre d'Etude de l'Energie Nucléaire,
Mol, Belgium

and

Michel Janowski[x] and M.S. Netrawali[xx]

Laboratoire de Morphologie Animale
Université Libre de Bruxelles,
Brussels, Belgium.

Abstract

Gamma- irradiation strongly inhibits in Acetabularia
mediterranea those processes which require the synthesis
of new "morphogenetic substances" (presumably m-RNA molecules). Labeling experiments with ^{3}H-5-uridine and ^{3}H -leu-
cine showed that transcription is inhibited, while translation continues at an almost normal rate in whole as well
as in anucleate cells.
With gamma-radiation cap formation and enzymes activity
(or synthesis) can be uncoupled. It is suggested that biochemical differentiation in the cytoplasm can go on in the
absence of morphological differentiation.

[x]Aspirant du Fonds National de la Recherche Scientifique.
[xx]Present address: Biochemistry and Food Technology Divi-
              sion, Bhabha Atomic Centre, Bombay 74, India.

255

Introduction

The unicellular giant alga Acetabularia mediterranea is very resistant to ionizing radiations (Bacq et al.1957; Six, 1958). This property may be due, at least in part, to the relative low (10^{-13}–10^{-12} g) DNA content of the nucleus (if the amount of DNA is related to the very large nuclear volume) (Dillard and Schweiger, 1969). The big nucleus ($\sim 10^{-3}$mm^3) of Acetabularia, during the vegetative stage is, in fact, Feulgen-negative. It was shown by Sparrow and Evans (1961), for a number of lower and higher plants, that the average amount of DNA per nucleus or per chromosome is correlated with the dose required to produce a lethal effect, the plants with low DNA content being the most radioresistant.

The aim of our work was to study the effect of gamma-radiation on the growth and differentiation of the algae. We report here the main results obtained in a series of biological and biochemical experiments.

I. Biological experiments

We have studied the effects of ^{60}Co gamma-radiation on the following processes:

a) cap formation in whole cells (fig.1) and in anucleate fragments (fig.2),

b) cap growth (fig.3 and 4),

c) cellular regeneration, from basal parts endowed of nucleus (fig.5),

d) cyst formation (fig.6).

The inhibition of cap formation increases in a linear way with the radiation doses. A dose of about $1.25 \cdot 10^5$ rad is required to stop completely cap formation (fig.7). However, at this and higher doses, the apical region of the cell appears altered, most frequently enlarged (fig.8).

Other modifications induced by different doses of radiation are:

a) loss of the whorls (fig.8),

b) abnormal enlargment of the whorls (fig.9 and 10),

c) ramification of the stalk (fig.7 and 11),

d) abnormal cap formation (fig.10 and 12).

The enlargement of the apical region suggests that the enzymes (mainly cell wall sugars hydrolysing and polymerising enzymes) normally involved in the construction of the cap's walls (cap formation) are still acting in the irradiated cell.

With gamma-radiation it seems thus possible to uncouple cap formation, which is a very complex event (Werz, 1965; Bonotto and Janowski, 1969), and enzyme activity. The high radioresistance of cap growth (fig.3 and 4) suggests equally that enzyme activity (or synthesis) is very little affected by radiation. Cellular regeneration (nucleate basal parts) and cyst formation are on the contrary more radiosensitive. This fact suggests that the cellular processes most affected by radiation are those which require a new synthesis of "morphogenetic substances" (presumably m-RNA molecules) by the primary nucleus (cellular regeneration) or by the secondary nuclei (cyst formation) in the cap (Hämmerling, 1934; Brachet, 1965; Hämmerling and Zetsche, 1966; Werz, 1968).

II. Biochemical experiments

The biological observations support the hypothesis that in Acetabularia, the gamma-rays inhibit more effectively the synthesis of new m-RNA molecules than the protein synthesis.

In order to check this hypothesis, we studied the effect of gamma-radiation on the incorporation of ^{3}H-5-uridine and of ^{3}H-leucine into the RNA and proteins respectively. The main results obtained in these experiments (fig.14) completely confirmed our hypothesis: RNA synthesis (transcription) is strongly inhibited by radiation, while protein synthesis (translation) is not or only little affected; no difference was observed between whole and anucleate cells. Parallel experiments showed, moreover, that ^{3}H-thymidine incorporation into the DNA was strongly inhibited by gamma-radiation (Netrawali, unpublished results; Bonotto and Kirchmann, in press, a).

III. Discussion

Gamma- irradiated Acetabularia cells, in which RNA (and DNA) synthesis is strongly inhibited, continue to perform protein synthesis at an almost normal rate. These results support the current hypothesis that, in Acetabularia, stable m-RNA molecules are stored in the cytoplasm (see for a review : Brachet, 1968). They suggest also that these supposed m-RNA molecules are particularly radioresistant. We can not exclude, however, the possibility of a new radioresistant synthesis of m-RNA molecules in the irradiated cells.

Translation in gamma-irradiated cells is probably performed on pre-existing ribosomes, since gamma-radiation strongly inhibits the synthesis of new ribosomes (Bonotto and Kirchmann, in press, a). Results obtained by treating the algae with actinomycin D or rifampicin support this hypothesis : protein synthesis continue almost normally, while RNA and ribosomes synthesis are strongly inhibited (Bonotto and Kirchmann, 1969). Pre-existing stable m-RNA molecules, if they exist in Acetabularia, seem thus display a high resistance to gamma-radiation as well as to actinomycin D or to rifampicin.

These supposed m-RNA molecules, stored in the cytoplasm and/or in the chloroplasts and the mitochondria, must be, moreover, powerfully protected, perhaps in ribonucleoprotein particles or in stable polyribosomes. Temporal utilization of these stable m-RNA molecules is probably under cytoplasmic control.

The extensive work of Zetsche (1966 a,b; 1968) showed, in fact, that the genetic information for the differentiation (stalk and cap formation) of Acetabularia is realized under a regulatory mechanism which takes place at the level of translation.

Our biological and biochemical experiments shown that with gamma-radiation cap formation and enzyme activity (or synthesis) can be uncoupled. In fact, high doses of gamma-radiation, which prevent the initiation of the cap, have practically no or little influence on cap growth and protein synthesis. Similar results were obtained by Zetsche, Grieninger and Anders (this Symposium) with p-fluorophenylalanine: cap initiation was blocked, while

UDPG-pyrophosphorylase continued to be synthesized.

Gamma- irradiated Acetabularia, unable to form a cap, show frequently the apical region of the stalk enlarged or of spheroidal shape. These atipical structures may be due to an alteration of the localization of the hydrolytical enzymes (or perhaps of the corresponding messenger RNA's) at the apex of the cell (Bonotto, 1968, 1969). Our findings suggest that gamma-radiation may prevent cap formation by altering the ultrastructural organization of the apical region of the stalk. The initiation of cap formation seems thus to require, in order to be realized, an ordinate ultrastructural organization. The importance of the structural properties of the apex of the cell for the realization of morphogenesis was first emphasized by Werz (1965).

Gamma-radiation, like p-fluorophenylalanine (Zetsche, Grieninger and Anders, this Symposium),seems to prevent the morphological differentiation (cap formation) probably without affecting the biochemical differentiation of the cytoplasm. Thus the absence of cap formation does not necessarily signify an inhibition of the differentiation of the cytoplasm, at the biochemical level. This concept should be kept in mind, especially when only morphological data are recorded to study differentiation in Acetabularia.

Acknowledgements

This work has been supported by the "Fonds de la Recherche Scientifique Fondamentale Collective" and by Research Contract Euratom-U.L.B. 007-61-10 ABIB.

We are indebted to Prof. M.Errera (Brussels) and to Prof. P.Manil (Gembloux) for fruitful discussions. We thank Mrs Eliane Bonnijns-Van Gelder and Mr E.Fagniart, Mr L.Lateur and Mr G.Bas for the excellent technical help.

We thank Dr. F.Knüsel (CIBA, Basel, Switzerland) and Mr Walter B. Gall (MERCK SHARP & DOHME, Rahway, New Jersey, U.S.A.) for a generous gift of Rifampicin and of Actinomycin D respectively.

References

Z.M. Bacq, F. Vanderhaeghe, J. Damblon, M. Errera and A. Herve, Exp. Cell Res. 12, 639 (1957).

S. Bonotto, Protoplasma 66, 55 (1968).

S. Bonotto, Giorn. Bot. Ital. 103, 153 (1969).

S. Bonotto, A. Goffeau, M. Janowski, T. Vanden Driessche and J. Brachet, Biochim. Biophys. Acta 174, 704 (1969).

S. Bonotto and M. Janowski, Bull.Soc.roy.Bot. Belgique 102, 257 (1969).

S. Bonotto and R. Kirchmann, Bull.Soc.roy.Bot. Belgique, in press, a.

S. Bonotto and R. Kirchmann, Bull.Soc.roy.Bot. Belgique, in press, b.

S. Bonotto and R. Kirchmann, Congresso Società Botanica Italiana, Siena 20-24 Ottobre 1969. Riassunti delle Comunicazioni Scientifiche, p. 4.

J. Brachet, Progress Biophys. Mol. Biol. 15, 97 (1965).

J. Brachet, Current Topics Develop. Biol. 3, 1 (1968).

W.L. Dillard and H.G. Schweiger, Protoplasma 67, 87 (1969).

J. Hämmerling, Wilhelm Roux' Archiv für Entwicklungsmechanik der Organismen 131, 1 (1934).

J. Hämmerling and K. Zetsche, Umschau 15, 489 (1966).

E. Six, Z. Naturforschg 13b, 6 (1958).

A.H. Sparrow and H.J. Evans, Brookhaven Symposia in Biology 14, 76 (1961).

G. Werz, Brookhaven Symposia in Biology 18, 185 (1965).

G. Werz, Protoplasma 65, 349 (1968).

K. Zetsche, Planta (Berl.) 68, 240 (1966a).

K. Zetsche, Z. Naturforschg 21b, 375 (1966b).

K. Zetsche, Z. Naturforschg 23b, 369 (1968).

K. Zetsche, G. Grieninger and J. Anders, this Symposium.

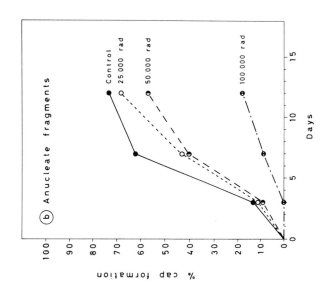

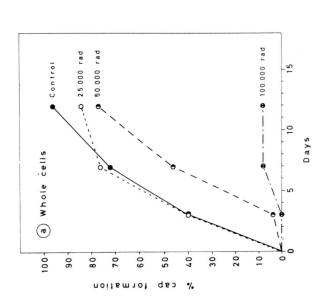

Fig. 1 and 2   Effect of radiation on cap formation in the presence and in the absence of the nucleus.

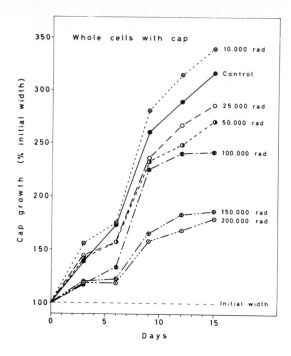

Fig. 3 Effect of radiation on cap growth:
this process is very radioresistant; even
doses, which completely inhibit cell regeneration and cap formation (150 - 200 000 rad)
still allow a certain development of the
initiated cap.

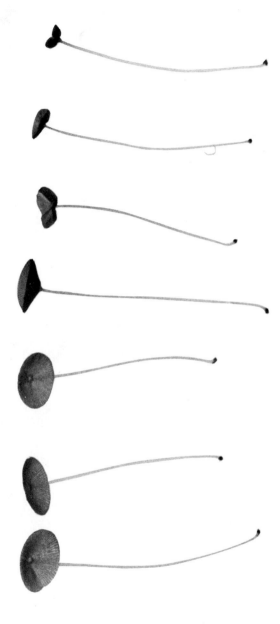

Fig. 4 Effect of radiation on cap growth. From left to right : Control and cells irradiated with 10 000, 25 000, 50 000, 100 000, 150 000 and 200 000 rad respectively.

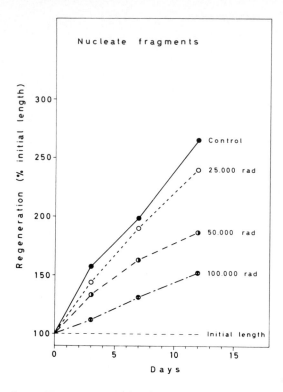

Fig. 5 Effect of radiation on cellular regeneration: basal fragments 5 mm long, with nucleus, were irradiated 48 h after cutting off the stalk. This process is more radiosensitive than cap formation or cap growth.

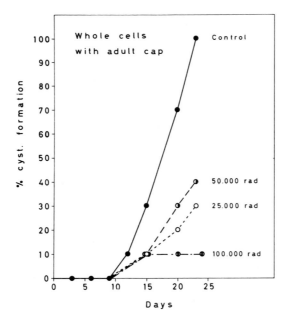

Fig. 6 Cyst formation is particularly radiosensitive: relative low doses (25 – 50 000 rad) of radiation strongly inhibit (60–70%) cyst formation, but not the migration of the cytoplasm into the cap's lodges.

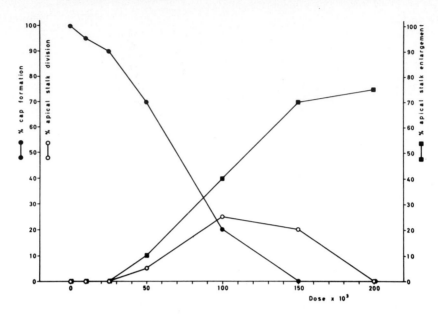

Fig. 7   This figure shows that a dose of
about $1.25 \cdot 10^5$ rad (extrapolated value)
is required to stop completely cap
formation in whole cells. The figure
shows also the induction of stalk
division and of stalk enlargement
(23 days after the irradiation).

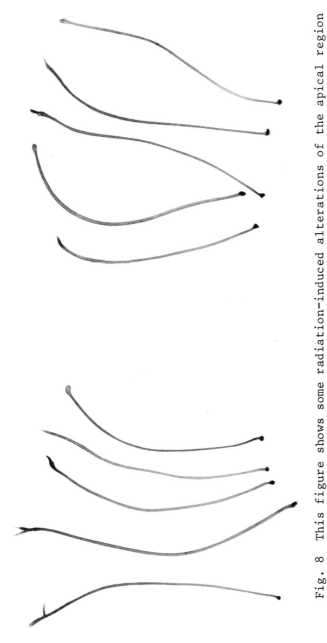

Fig. 8 This figure shows some radiation-induced alterations of the apical region in whole cells. The cells were irradiated with 150 000 (left) or with 200 000 (right) rad.
The picture was taken 23 days after the irradiation, when the controls (not shown here) already presented well developed caps.

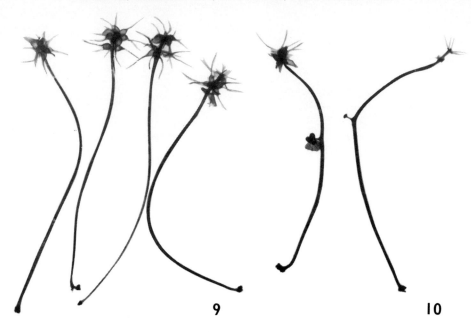

9   **10**

Fig. 9 Four <u>Acetabularia</u> whole cells showing radiation-induced abnormal enlargement of the
whorls.
The cells were irradiated (100 000 rad) before cap formation.

Fig. 10 Two <u>Acetabularia</u> whole cells showing radiation-induced abnormal morphogenesis : abnor-
mal enlargement of the whorls and abnormal
lateral cap formation.
The cells were irradiated (125 000 rad) before cap formation.

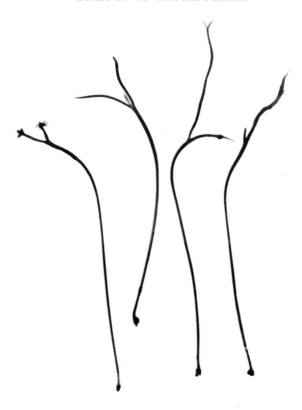

Fig. 11   Whole <u>Acetabularia</u> cells showing
radiation-induced stalk division.
The cells were irradiated (100 000 rad)
before cap formation.

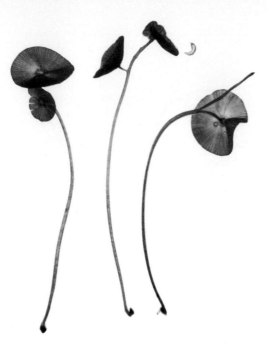

Fig. 12   Whole <u>Acetabularia</u> cells showing radiation-
induced stalk division and some abnormal
caps.
The cells were irradiated (75 000 rad)
before cap formation.

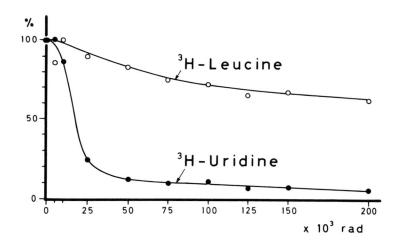

Fig. 13   This figure shows that increasing doses of
radiation strongly inhibit the incorporation
of ^{3}H-5- uridine into the RNA, while the incorporation of ^{3}H-leucine into the proteins
seems little affected. 10 whole cells (stage
4, S_{30}, W_3 : Bonotto and Kirchmann, in press,
b) were incubated 60 min in the presence of
25 µCi/ml of ^{3}H-5-uridine or of ^{3}H-leucine,
45 min after the irradiation, and processed
as previously described in Bonotto <u>et al</u>.
(1969).

ignorant of what we are really doing when we cut an Acetabularia into two : would algae grown in the Mediterranean
always behave like the carefully nursed algae cultivated
in laboratories under artificial conditions ? If illumination is a factor which could and should be rather easy to
control, so that standardized conditions of intensity,
wavelength and periodicity could be adopted, earth extract
remains a variable : we know that the earth extract from
the Naples volcanic area kindly sent to us by K. Beth,
ensures better growth than the one obtained from our heavy
flemish soils, but we do not know why. It is to be hoped
that, as a result of this Symposium, exchange of strains
and of technical information, will become more and more
frequent.

The danger of bacterial contamination, especially
in biochemical experiments requiring the use of radioactive
isotopes, is now present in all our minds : no experiment,
in this field, will be really convincing unless it is proved by microbiological techniques and by electron microscopy that bacterial contamination is negligible or absent.
The ultimate aim is, of course, to obtain sterile cultures
in chemically defined media (earth extract is, of course,
very complex and we found, for instance, that it contains
all the usual aminoacids) : the difficulties to be overcome before we reach this goal are great, due to the length
(several months) of the reproductive cycle, the inhibitory
effects of many antibiotics on several biochemical processes occuring in the alga and a puzzling fact that I observed long ago (Brachet, 1958) : the algae "do not like"
normal aminoacids, purines or pyrimidines and, in general,
fare better in the presence of their analogs. The probable
reason is the difficulty of keeping the medium sterile when
it contains normal metabolites.

Other technical points have their importance, for
instance the precautions taken in order to inhibit the
degradation of macromolecules, the Mg^{++} content of the
medium, etc. But even such trivial things as the method
used for cutting the algae, the localization of the cut
(very near the nucleus or in the lower third of the stalk),
the time allowed for repair, etc. may be very important :
I have observed (unpublished) that sectioning the alga
can produce, on the next day, a reduction of the nuclear
volume of 100 times or more. The effects on

274

the nucleus of the "surgical shock" are greatest when
the section is made very close to the rhizoids : in fact,
under these conditions, the nucleolus loses much of its
basophilia : it is probable that such nucleate fragments
are temporarily paralyzed and that they behave more like
anucleate than nucleate fragments.

2. Present conclusions and some problems for the future.

Not much can be added to the fundamental work of
J. Hämmerling and his school (in particular, K.Beth)about
the role of the nucleus in the production of the species-
specific morphogenetic substances which control regeneration. In the absence of new data about morphogenesis
(except those given by S. Bonotto and his coll. on the effects of ionizing radiations), the general discussion,
about the purely biological phenomena remained somewhat
byzantine : we learned from K. Beth that Acetabularia mediterranea is not the right name for this organism, according to the rules of taxonomy. I hope that these rules
will not be obeyed, because it took me a long time to
discover that Spisula is the good old Mactra, that the
Strongylocentrotus on which my father was working 50 years
ago is a Paracentrotus, that the Rana fusca of the embryo-
logists is in fact Rana temporaria, etc. We already have
so many problems with Acetabularia that we should not add
to the existing complications by changing its name.
Another byzantine question came up several times:
is Acetabularia a cell or an organism ? Granting that it
has everything which is characteristic of a green plant
cell, I personally think that it is somewhat more than
that, because of the existence of a reproductive cycle
(formation of gametes and zygotes). I do not like to
hear an egg called a cell, since it has the potentialities of producing, even by parthenogenesis, an adult of
the utmost complication. But this is a matter of taste
and it is now time to go into more important questions.
At the purely biological level, many important con-
tributions have been brought to the Symposium by various

participants. Certain disputed points about the formation of the gametes and their fusion have been clarified by J.C.W. Crawley's studies with the electron microscope, while several theoretical questions concerning growth, cap formation and dormancy of the cysts have been raised by K. Beth. The ultrastructure of the alga has been studied by several participants (G. Werz, S. Puiseux-Dao, M. Boloukhère) : thanks to their efforts, we now know much more about the fine structure of the chloroplasts and the mitochondria, including the localization of their DNA's. The extensive work of M. Boloukhère, who studied in detail the ultrastructure of the alga, at the unicellular and multicellular stages, and under various experimental conditions (darkness, enucleation) will remain a very useful basis for further experimental and biochemical work. The electron micrographs shown on the screen were very beautiful , despite the technical difficulties presented by this organism which lives in sea water, has a large internal vacuole of acid pH (J.C.W. Crawley, 1963) and is surrounded by a thick and complex cell wall : they were a real pleasure for the eyes and a relief, for myself at any rate, from the long succession of sucrose gradients and other diagrams which we saw.

At the molecular biology level, nobody doubted that the "central dogma" (DNA $\longrightarrow$ RNA $\longrightarrow$ protein) holds true for Acetabularia as well as for E.coli. But everybody agreed that Acetabularia, even if it is just a cell, is somewhat more complicated than an E.coli: it has chloroplasts (which very much attract biochemists), it has a delicate ultrastructure which changes during the cell cycle and under various experimental conditions (as shown by S. Puiseux-Dao, G. Werz and M. Boloukhère), it can form cysts and gametes in a cap which has a complex and species-specific morphology. Therefore more information would be expected to be contained in the nuclear DNA of an Acetabularia than in a bacterial chromosome.

In the following, a number of questions will be asked regarding successively nuclear DNA, cytoplasmic DNA, transcription and translation in Acetabularia.

a) Nuclear DNA. The only quantitative data we have about the DNA content of the Acetabularia nucleus comes from the work of G. Werz : using the Feulgen reaction and a cytophotometric method, he found 10^{-13} gr/nucleus in

the diploid zygote. But this measurement, in view of the
uncertainties of the cytophotometric method when it is used
for quantitative purposes, should be checked by a more direct, biochemical approach. Measurement of the DNA content
of a known number of gametes is no good, since the gametes
possess chloroplasts. The only way seems to be to sacrifice
enough algae for isolating the nuclei, and to measure their
DNA content quantitatively by a refined method such as that
of Edström (1964). Such an experiment is badly needed, since we completely lose the track of the nuclear DNA as soon
as the zygote nucleus begins to grow (even staining with
^{3}H-actinomycin, which is a more refined method than the
Feulgen reaction, does not give a clearcut answer about the
localization of DNA in the enlarged nucleus.
Therefore, we do not yet know whether the large nucleus of
the full grown alga still contains the same amount of DNA
as the zygote nucleus : on the basis of the cytochemical
tests, one would come to the paradoxical conclusion that
this nucleus, which contains enough information to produce
a cap, has no DNA at all ! Of course, we do not believe
that this is so ; but belief and rigorous scientific demonstration are two different things. The paucity of DNA
in the large Acetabularia nucleus suggests that no endopo-
lyploidy occurs during the growth of the alga ; but we are
not sure that the nuclear DNA is never replicated until the
big vegetative nucleus breaks down.
        This nuclear breakdown raises other questions : we
know, from Hämmerling's work (1934, a,b,c) that this process is controled by cytoplasmic factors linked to the age
of the plant (grafting of an old stalk on a nucleate half
induces nuclear breakdown, removal of cytoplasm prior to
cap formation inhibits it). What could be the chemical
nature of these cytoplasmic factors ? Is there a synthesis or activation of DNA polymerase, when the DNA of the
decaying large nucleus begins to replicate in order to
form the secondary nuclei ? The situation is reminescent
of that studied by Gurdon (1962) when he injected old nuclei into the young cytoplasm of anucleate unfertilized
Xenopus eggs. Would, as in that case, synthesis of r-RNA
be repressed when the primary nucleus (which has a huge
nucleolus) breaks down ? In other words, would there be,
at that time, a cytoplasmically regulated shift from r-
RNA to DNA synthesis ? The possibilities offered by

Acetabularia for the study of events which occur after
nuclear breakdown have been badly overlooked so far.
In fact, we do not even know with certainty when and where
meiosis occurs in Acetabularia and we have no idea at all
about the length of the various phases of the cell cycle
in the secondary nuclei. No attempt has been made to
synchronize cell division in the latter and we cannot
guess what would be the effect on morphogenesis if one
succeeded in doing so.

     b) Cytoplasmic DNA. We are, at least, certain of
its existence: Acetabularia contains easily measurable
amounts of DNA, localized in the chloroplasts and in
the mitochondria. The exact density of these two DNA's,
in CsCl density gradients, remains controversial, probably because the mitochondrial fraction is often contaminated by microorganisms. Nevertheless, it now seems to
be generally accepted that mitochondrial DNA has a higher
density (1.714 gr/cm3) and is present in much smaller
amounts than chloroplastic DNA (density 1.704). It is also
agreed that chloroplastic DNA is made of fibres which can
be as long as 28 µ, but it is not known whether mitochondrial DNA is a circular molecule (G. Werz, B. Green et
al., in this Symposium). The fact that prolonged darkness
reduces the light DNA peak (1.704) and that ethidium bromide produces, in a short time, the disappearance of the
heavy one (1.714) lends further support to their identi-
fication as chloroplastic and mitochondrial DNA's respectively. The effectiveness of ethidium bromide in suppres-
sing the mitochondrial DNA peak (S. Limbosch and V. Heilporn) raises the interesting question of a possible role
of mitochondrial DNA in morphogenesis : cap formation is
quickly suppressed by ethidium bromide in both nucleate
and anucleate fragments (J. Brachet 1968; V. Heilporn and
S. Limbosch, 1969) and the reasons for this inhibition
might deserve a careful biochemical analysis.

     What is the function of chloroplastic DNA ? There
is no doubt that it can be both transcribed (H.G. Schweiger and S. Berger, 1964) and translated (A. Goffeau and
J. Brachet, 1965). The proteins which are synthesized
under the control of chloroplastic DNA are the structural
proteins of the chloroplasts ; the other chloroplastic
proteins, including the enzymes required for photosynthesis are probably synthesized under the control of nuclear

genes. It is not known whether chloroplastic DNA has sequences in common with nuclear DNA in Acetabularia ; nothing is known either about the nature of the RNA's synthesized on the chloroplastic DNA template. These are fascinating problems, which require mass isolation of mitochondria and chloroplasts from Acetabularia for their
solution.

How much DNA is there in an Acetabularia chloroplast ? The answers vary, by a factor of 10, and consequently so does the estimate for the number of proteins
which could be   coded by   the chloroplastic DNA template. Such estimates should be regarded as maximal and
highly hypothetical, since the possibility of gene redun-
dancy in chloroplastic DNA cannot be excluded on an a
priori basis.

Finally, there is no doubt that chloroplastic DNA
can be replicated in the absence of the nucleus, since
both the number of chloroplasts and the DNA content markedly increase in the absence of the nucleus (D. Shephard,
1965, V. Heilporn and J. Brachet, 1966). But the increase
in number of the chloroplasts is markedly slower in anucleate than in nucleate fragments : something which is
needed for the division of the chloroplasts is missing
in the former and must be provided by the nucleus. We have
no idea whatsoever about the chemical nature of these
"factors" of nuclear origin. Nor do we know anything about
the enzymatic equipment for DNA synthesis (kinases, syn-
thetase, polymerase, etc.) present in chloroplasts isolated from Acetabularia.

c) RNA synthesis. Already in 1959, I made the sug-
gestion that morphogenesis is controled, in Acetabularia,
by an RNA which would originate from the nucleus and migrate to the tip of the alga where it would retain the information it has received from the nucleus for a considerable time. Shortly afterwards, the name messenger RNA
(mRNA) was coined for the short lived RNA molecules which
carry to the bacterial ribosomes the information they need
for the synthesis of specific proteins. It is now admitted
that the half life of m-RNA's is highly variable. The
hypothesis that a very stable m-RNA, produced by the nucleus, is the biochemical counterpart of Hämmerling's
"morphogenetic substances" remains a basic concept for all
those who are engaged in research on Acetabularia.

However, it should be stressed that the situation remains far from satisfactory in this respect for the time being. A first point to be made is that it is most unlikely that we should think in terms of one single m-RNA : we know, from the work presented here by K. Zetsche and by G. Werz, that many enzymes involved in cell wall formation are synthesized in larger amounts at the time of cap formation. The same is true for acid (Triplett et al. 1965) and alkaline phosphatases (Spencer and Harris, 1964), two enzymes of unknown function in the alga. Probably many other enzymes, as yet unstudied, also show considerable increases in activity when caps form, whether the nucleus is present or not. This means that there must exist in the alga a whole array of stable m-RNA molecules, coding for the synthesis of many different proteins. Or, but this seems much less likely, we have to think in terms of a giant polycistronic m-RNA molecule. Are these m-RNA's synthesized by an operon, which could be switched on and off, as in bacteria, by an operator gene ? Only an analysis, in relation with time, of the synthesis of many enzymes could give an answer. One would rather expect a negative one, in view of the fact that, in slime-molds, where several enzymes involved in cell-wall formation are synthesized at given stages of the biological cycle, there is no evidence so far for the operon concept (Sussman, 1965).

Thus, to say that "the cap is formed by a stable m-RNA" is an obvious oversimplification : one thing that we need is more insight into the molecular mechanisms of cap formation (tridimensional structure of the cap proteins and polysaccharides, possible selfassembly of preformed subunits, etc.). This would certainly be a rewarding task for biophysicists and would bring important information to the biologists.

The nearest approach to an experimental demonstration of the existence of stable m-RNA molecules in Acetabularia comes from the work, done in my laboratory, by F. Farber et al. (1968): she was able to show that whole algae contain template RNA's (i.e. RNA's which are able to support in vitro the synthesis of polypeptide chains in an acellular bacterial system). While template activity is one of the attributes of m-RNA's, identity of the latter with template RNA's cannot be accepted unless it

is demonstrated that no other RNA fraction extracted from
the cell has a template activity. This was not done in
Farber et al.'s work (1968) ; but nevertheless, an interesting discovery was made : in contrast to the above
mentioned enzymes, the amount of template RNA decreases
when the caps begin to form. It looks as if this particular kind of RNA, like the morphogenetic substances,
would be used up when the enzymes required for cap formation are synthesized. Unfortunately, certain basic questions have not yet been answered : is template RNA also
present in anucleate fragments ? How does it behave (stability or degradation) when the two kinds of fragments
are compared ? Is it localized, like the morphogenetic
substances, along an apico-basal decreasing gradient ?
Is its formation, in nucleate halves, inhibited by actinomycin ? Clearcut answers to these vital questions might,
ultimately, enable us to identify Farber et al.'s (1968)
template RNA with the still hypothetical stable m-RNA of
nuclear origin of Acetabularia. However, the full demonstration of the hypothesis will not be given until we can
isolate, in highly purified form, RNA preparations which,
after injection into a basal fragment of the stalk (which
very seldom regenerates) will form a species-specificic
cap!   Much more is known about chloroplastic RNA and
chloroplastic ribosomes, which undergo extensive synthesis
in the absence of the nucleus (the RNA content of anucleate fragments doubles within a week, as a result of chloroplastic RNA synthesis). Extensive studies about the synthesis of the chloroplastic ribosomes and their sub-units
will be found in the reports of W.L. Dillard and M. Janowski in the present book. Two findings deserve particular
attention : the formation of polysomes in anucleate halves,
and the existence of a 15 S RNA endowed with unusual stability, since it remains detectable for more than 3 months
in anucleate as well as in nucleate halves. What could be
the origin of the m-RNA which is synthesized and binds to
ribosomes in the absence of the nucleus ? We do not yet
know, the answer ; but the fact that the synthesis of this
RNA is greatly enhanced when algae kept for some time in
the dark are illuminated suggests that it might be of
chloroplastic origin. But one cannot exclude a more fan-
ciful hypothesis (once suggested privately to me by Prof.
S. Spiegelman), invoking the presence of a viral RNA in

the algae, despite the fact that so far electron microscopy has never detected any viral-like inclusion. The
existence of a very stable form of RNA is important, because it shows that certain RNA species are not easily
degraded inside the living algae. This finding adds to the
credibility of the stable m-RNA story; however, the stable
15 S RNA studied by Janowski cannot be the elusive m-RNA
supposed to be responsible for cap formation, since it can
be synthesized in the absence of the nucleus.

A better place to look for m-RNA production, in
Acetabularia, would probably be the nucleus. But we know
next to nothing about the RNA's synthesized by this nucleus : there has been no report so far on the base composition or the sedimentation constants of the RNA's in either isolated nuclei, or nuclei dissected out of algae
submitted to pulses of various lengths of time with suitable precursors. Such a kinetic analysis of nuclear RNA
synthesis is badly needed and should be feasible : what
has been achieved with Chironomus salivary gland cell
nuclei must be possible with Acetabularia nuclei. All that
is required is patience, care and utilization of the ultra-
micromethods which enabled Baltus et al. (1968) to measure
the base composition of nucleolar and nuclear sap RNA's in
Acetabularia. The results obtained were interesting enough
to deserve a continuation of the work : nuclear sap RNA
was found to be rich in uracil, a finding which is becoming more and more significant since we know that many nuclei contain large, uracil rich RNA molecules, which are
not found in the cytoplasm and which presumably play a
role in the regulation of genetic activity. The RNA present in the huge nucleolus has also a puzzling base composition : it is not of the usual G + C rich type, but
DNA-like. One might wonder whether, in this alga, where
DNA must supply a lot of information in order to control
morphogenesis, DNA-like m-RNA molecules (m-RNA's perhaps)
are not temporarily stored in the nucleolus. Strangely
enough, it has never been possible to isolate clean ribosomes from the cytoplasm of Acetabularia, so that the base
compositions of r-RNA and nucleolar RNA could not be compared. Ribosomes exist, of course, in the cytoplasm of the
alga, as shown by electron microscopy. But we do not know
what happens to them and to their RNA's after enucleation,
except for the fact that ribosome-like particles can still

be seen, by electron microscopy, in the cytoplasm of
anucleate fragments (M. Boloukhère, this Symposium).

d) Regulation of protein synthesis in the presence or the absence of the nucleus.

A brief comparison between the anucleate fragments
of sea urchin eggs and those of Acetabularia might have
some interest. Unfertilized sea urchin eggs can be cut into two halves by gradient centrifugation; neither the nucleate, nor the anucleate halves display protein synthetic
activities. But, after parthenogenetic stimulation by
treatment with hypertonic sea water, both fragments quickly and strongly incorporate aminoacids into their proteins.
It can be shown that protein synthesis, in both halves, is
mediated by polysomes. The conclusion seems clear : as in
Acetabularia, unfertilized sea urchin eggs must contain
masked, stable m-RNA molecules, which combine with the
pre-existing ribosomes in order to form active polysomes
after parthenogenetic activation (see Brachet, 1966, for
a more complete review of the metabolism of anucleate fragments of sea urchin eggs). Another similarity between sea
urchin eggs and Acetabularia is the presence of cytoplasmic DNA in both : in sea urchin eggs, it is localized in
the mitochondria (and possibly in the yolk platelets, as
shown by Pikò et al. 1967). There is some evidence that,
like chloroplastic DNA in Acetabularia, it is capable of
replication in the absence of the nucleus. But there is
one big difference between Acetabularia and sea urchin
eggs : while the former can produce caps in the absence
of the nucleus, the second can, at best, start an irregular and abortive cleavage. All they can do is to form as-
ters and furrows, and there is no true morphogenesis (not
even formation of cilia and hatching). In fact, there is
fairly good evidence for the view that the aster rays result from the self assembly of the pre-existing sub-units
of the microtubules and that contractile proteins already
exist in the cortex. There is no evidence, so far, that
the proteins which are synthesized immediately after ferti-
lization or parthenogenesis play a role in the abortive
cleavage displayed by the activated anucleate halves.
The nature of these proteins and their possible role still
remain completely unknown. But the very existence of their

synthesis in the absence of the nucleus shows that <u>controls</u>
<u>at the translational level</u> exist in sea urchin eggs <u>as well</u>
<u>as in Acetabularia</u>. The case of the sea urchin egg is cer-
tainly not unique, since it has been shown that amphibian
eggs can cleave and produce proteins under conditions in
which no RNA synthesis is possible (experiments of actinomycin micro-injection by Brachet et al. 1964b).

Let us go back, after this parenthesis, to <u>Acetabu-</u>
<u>laria</u>, which differs so strikingly from sea urchin eggs by
the presence of chloroplasts and by its much higher potentialities for morphogenesis in the absence of the nucleus. The presence of large amounts of chloroplastic DNA
and the already discussed capacity for independent RNA and
protein synthesis of isolated chloroplasts makes conclusions about the respective role of controls at the transcription and translation levels difficult : even if a
given protein (an enzyme, for instance) is synthesized in
the absence of the nucleus and is found in the cytoplasm,
it is difficult to prove that it was not synthesized in
the chloroplasts (under the control of chloroplastic DNA)
and transferred to the cytoplasm.

Since a number of enzymes have been studied in
<u>Acetabularia</u>, we are in a better position than in the case
of sea urchin eggs concerning the synthesis of specific
proteins in the absence of the nucleus. Many enzymes, most
of them chloroplastic, have been found to increase several
fold in anucleate fragments of the algae (see Brachet and
Lang, for a review (1963).

One of the most interesting among these enzymes is
UDPG pyrophosphorylase, which has been so carefully studied by K. Zetsche : not only the activity of this enzyme
increases at the time of cap formation, but its distribution along the apico-basal gradient is the same as that of
the "morphogenetic substances". However, the use of an
inhibitor of cap formation (p-fluoro-phenylalanine) shows
that it is possible to dissociate enzyme synthesis from
morphogenesis : the synthesis of the enzyme occurs even
when caps are not produced.

Interesting effects of various inhibitors on the
synthesis of the same enzyme, and on the overall synthesis of proteins have also been described by K. Zetsche in
this Symposium. The effect of these inhibitors of protein
synthesis (puromycin, cycloheximide, chloramphenicol) on

morphogenesis have also been studied, as well as those of
RNA synthesis inhibitors (Brachet et al. 1964a, Zetsche,
1965) : the results were essentially the same in the two
laboratories.

But a word of caution about the interpretation of
such biological experiments is necessary. We have studied
(Bonotto et al. 1969) the effects of four inhibitors of
protein synthesis (puromycin, cycloheximide, chloramphenicol and tetracycline) on morphogenesis, protein and RNA
synthesis in nucleate and anucleate halves of Acetabularia;
isolated chloroplasts were compared, as far as protein
synthesis goes, with the living fragments of the alga.
It was found that tetracycline and chloramphenicol strongly inhibit protein synthesis in the isolated chloroplasts,
while cycloheximide had no effect. But when the antibiotics were tested on living algae, both the uptake of aminoacids and their incorporation into protein were blocked
by all four inhibitors. The inhibition of protein synthesis was of the same order of magnitude, in both nucleate
and anucleate fragments, for chloroplastic and non chloroplastic proteins. Furthermore, even RNA synthesis in vivo
was strongly inhibited, already after 2 days of treatment,
by all the inhibitors except cycloheximide : again, there
was no difference between chloroplastic and cytoplasmic
RNA's. On the other hand, the antibiotics which, in vitro,
act on cytoplasmic polysomes (puromycin and cycloheximide)
and those which inhibit protein synthesis in isolated chloroplasts (chloramphenicol and tetracycline) have entirely
different effects on morphogenesis: the former inhibit
regeneration, reversibly in nucleate fragments, irreversi-
bly in anucleate ones ; the second (like actinomycin) allow cap formation in anucleate fragments, but slow down
their growth. The simplest interpretation of these biological experiments would be that regeneration is completely stopped when cytoplasmic protein synthesis is inhibited,
while caps can be formed, but grow slowly, when chloroplastic protein synthesis is blocked. The biochemical experiments presented above show that such an easy explanation
cannot be true since the so-called "specific" inhibitors
of protein synthesis quickly interfere with both chloroplastic and cytoplasmic RNA synthesis. This word of caution does not hold solely for Acetabularia, but should
be kept in mind by the "cytopharmacologists". To be

285

complete, it might be added that rifampicin inhibits quickly (in 90 min.) and strongly (65%-75%) RNA synthesis in Acetabularia, without affecting protein, DNA (chloroplastic and mitochondrial) synthesis and photosynthesis (Bonotto, Janowski, Vanden Driessche and Brachet, 1968). Nevertheless, the biological effects are not very impressive : there is only a general retardation of growth and of cap formation in both nucleate and anucleate halves.

These experiments, as well as the earlier ones of Zetsche (1965) with puromycin, show that the alga (or at least, the nucleate and anucleate fragments) should be considered as a whole, and that chloroplasts and "cytoplasm" can only be separated for operational purposes (in particular, for biochemical work).

The elegant experiments, reported by H.G. Schweiger in this Symposium, on the effects of inter-specific grafts of nucleate and anucleate fragments on the control of malate dehydrogenase synthesis point in the same direction : the isozyme pattern is nucleus-dependent. The exact localization of the enzyme (chloroplastic or mitochondrial) has been the object of controversies during the Symposium; it is to be hoped that new experiments will solve this question. But, the major point, i.e. that the synthesis of some enzymes localized in cytoplasmic organelles is controlled by the nucleus, remains undisputed.

We have tried to attack the important problem of the regulation of specific enzyme synthesis from a different angle (Brachet and Lievens, 1968) ; the experiments have been done several years ago, but publication in a russian journal has been delayed for no known reason. We worked on acid phosphatase, because this enzyme had already been studied in our laboratory and asked ourselves the following questions : since phosphatases are repressible enzymes in many cases, would removal of the end product of the reaction (inorganic phosphate : Pi) from the medium stimulate enzymatic activity ? Since, as we had found earlier, (Triplett et al., 1965) there are 5 detectable isozymes of acid phosphatase, would the activity of all of them be regulated simultaneously ? Would regulation of the various isozymes be regulated in the same way in nucleate and anucleate fragments of Acetabularia ? To answer these questions, we have cultivated whole algae, nucleate and anucleate halves in a Pi poor medium

and followed the activity of the 3 main isozymes of acid
phosphatase. Unexpectedly, the activity of the isozymes
decreased, in all cases, after a few days of culture in
the Pi deficient medium. The reasons for this paradoxical
result could be understood when the fate of the polyphosphate pool was followed during the culture : there is a
marked and progressive breakdown of the large polyphosphates when the algae are placed in the Pi poor medium,
so that the internal Pi concentration of the algae remains
normal. After 10-12 days, in the phosphate deficient medium, phosphatase activity remains constant for a few
days. At that time, the activity increases considerably
(becoming higher than the initial value) in the whole algae and the nucleate halves ; this increase does not occur
in the anucleate fragments. Electrophoretic analysis
shows that the proportion of the isozymes changes independently from each other. The experiments, which deserve
further analysis, clearly indicate that certain regulatory mechanisms for enzyme activity or synthesis which exist
in nucleate algae are missing when the nucleus has been
removed. It would be premature to go further and to try
to build a model which would explain these facts until
further information has been obtained in this subject.

e. More about the partial dependence of the chloroplasts on the nucleus.

Although isolated chloroplasts are, as shown in
this Symposium, capable of protein synthesis (A. Goffeau)
and of perfect photosynthesis, which requires the harmo-
nious functioning of many enzymes (D. Shephard), they are
dependent upon the nucleus for their multiplication : the
early finding of D. Shephard (1965b) that the increase in
chloroplast number is slower in anucleate than in nucleate
fragments has been made much more precise by the thorough
analysis by S. Puiseux-Dao of the structure and ultrastructure of the chloroplasts : the existence of "plastidial units" , involved in carbohydrate synthesis and in
chloroplast reproduction has been well demonstrated by
her work. Her careful observations agree with the view
that the chloroplasts require "something" of nuclear origin in order to be biochemically fully active. What remains unclear, however, is the chemical nature of the

287

polysaccharide synthesized by the <u>Acetabularia</u> chloroplasts : it might be starch, or inulin, or a mixture of both. Although this point is of minor importance, it is to be hoped that it will soon be clarified.

But it is perhaps in the studies on the <u>circadian rhythms</u>, in nucleate and anucleate fragments of <u>Acetabularia</u>, that the delicacy of the nucleo-chloroplastic interrelations appear most clearly : anucleate fragments of <u>Acetabularia</u> retain their circadian rhythm of photosynthesis for a considerable period, as was first shown by G. Richter (1963). But, as demonstrated by Schweiger, Wallraff and Schweiger, (1964), who grafted together nucleate and anucleate fragments having different rhythms, the "clock" is set by the nucleus. No less impressive are T. Vanden Driessche's experiments (1967) : she grafted nucleate fragments from normal algae to anucleate stalks from strains which had lost their rhythm of photosynthetic capacity and found that the circadian rhythm of photosynthesis is restored. The reciprocal experiment showed that grafting the rhizoïd of an "arythmic" alga on the green stalk of a normal alga induces the loss of the circadian rhythm. Thus a purely chloroplastic function (photosynthesis) is controlled, so far as rhythmicity goes, by the nucleus. As can be seen in T. Vanden Driessche's contribution to this Symposium, there exist many circadian rhythms (polysaccharide content, RNA and ATP content, shape of the chloroplast, etc.) besides the one of governing photosynthetic activity in <u>Acetabularia</u>. Their interrelationships is now being worked out. Furthermore, experiments with inhibitors of RNA and protein synthesis suggest that m—RNA's of nuclear origin play a central role in these circadian rhythms. Although the latter are affected by the inhibitors in the same way as morphogenesis, it is difficult, for the time being, to decide whether they have a direct influence on morphogenesis itself : the fact that "arythmic" algae can form caps is a matter of concern in this respect.

f) Effects of radiations on morphogenesis

The effects of monochromatic blue and red light have been studied by H. Clauss and G. Richter : since there were major points of disagreement among them, the non-specialists will remain "in the dark" for the time being.

But there is no doubt that this kind of experiment might well become a very useful tool for future research on nucleocytoplasmic interactions in Acetabularia.

The Symposium was sponsored by Euratom and by the Centre of nuclear Energy (C.E.N) in Mol : it was fit to have a paper on the effects of ionizing radiations on Acetabularia, and this was done by S. Bonotto and his colleagues. Their experiments have confirmed the considerable radioresistance of both kinds of fragments, first described by Bacq et al. (1957). It was further shown that the irradiated algae often display anomalies of development (dichotomy, for instance, is rather frequent). Furthermore, the biochemical effects of the ionizing radiations were studied for the first time : inhibition of DNA, RNA and, to a lesser extent, protein synthesis was observed. Of special interest is the inhibition of DNA synthesis : since it occurs in anucleate as well as in nucleate halves, it seems clear that the replication of chloroplastic DNA is, like that of chromosomal DNA, sensitive to ionizing radiations.

There are some indications that the cysts are more radiosensitive than the still unicellular algae : this observation could be extremely important for the future since, in order to explore fully the possibilities given by Acetabularia, the obtention of mutants, suitable for genetical and refined biochemical analysis, is badly required. The long life cycle of the alga has so far prevented the initiation of studies of Acetabularia genetics : all efforts in order to speed up its development are valuable and might have important consequences.

3. Final words.

The Symposium has been successful because the scientists who attented it had many frank discussions, from which have arisen new ideas, new research programs and a sincere wish for collaboration. Private conversations, close contacts between participants did much for mutual understanding, not only of individuals, but even of Nations. For this reason, the Symposium has served, in its modest way, the great cause of Peace.

It is to be hoped that there will be other Symposia on Acetabularia, until Prof. Hämmerling's (whose absence was very much regretted) morphogenetic substances have been isolated in highly purified, if not crystalline, form. I hope that they will turn out to be a mixture of stable m-RNA molecules; but future research will certainly yield many surprises when we know more about this curious object, which was once humorously called an "animal honoris causa" by Prof. V. Hamburger.

References

Z. Bacq, F. Vanderhaeghe, J. Damblon, M. Errera and A. Herve (1957) Exptl. Cell Res. 12, 639.

E. Baltus, J.E. Edström, M. Janowski, J. Hanocq-Quertier, R. Tencer and J. Brachet (1968) Proc.natl.Acad.Sci. N.Y. 59, 406.

S. Bonotto, A. Goffeau, M. Janowski, T. Vanden Driessche and J. Brachet (1969) Biochim. Biophys. Acta 174, 704.

S. Bonotto, M. Janowski, T. Vanden Driessche and J. Brachet (1968) Arch. Intern. Physiol. Biochim. 76, 919.

J. Brachet (1958). Exptl. Cell Res. 14, 650.

J. Brachet (1959). Biological role of ribonucleic acids. Ed. Elsevier, Amsterdam.

J. Brachet (1966) Lunteren Symposium, pp. 330-343 Ed. Elsevier, Amsterdam.

J. Brachet, H. Denis and F. de Vitry (1964a) Developm. Biol. 9, 398.

J. Brachet, H. Denis and F. de Vitry (1964b) Developm. Biol. 9, 458.

J. Brachet and A. Lang (1963). Handbuch Pflanzenphysiol. 15, 1.

J. Brachet (1968). Nature 220, 488.

J. Brachet and A. Lievens (1968) Biokhimija, in the press.

J.C.W. Crawley (1963). Exptl. Cell Res. 32, 368.

W.L. Dillard and H.G. Schweiger (1969) Protoplasma 67, 87.

J.E. Edström (1964) in "Methods in Cell Physiology" vol. I, pp. 417-446 Ed. Prescott, Academic Press-New York.

F.E. Farber, M. Cape, M. Decroly and J. Brachet (1968) Proc. natl. Acad. Sci. N.Y. 61, 843.

A. Goffeau and J. Brachet (1965) Biochim. Biophys. Acta 95, 302.

J. Gurdon (1962) J. Embryol. exp. 10, 622.

J. Hammerling (1934a) Biol. Zbl. 59, 158.

J. Hämmerling (1934b) Naturwiss. 22, 829.

J. Hämmerling (1934c) Arch. Entwickl. Organ. Mech. 131, 1.

V. Heilporn and S. Limbosch (1969) Arch. int. Physiol. Bioch. 77, 383.

L. Pikó, A. Tyler and J. Vinograd (1967). Biol. Bull. 132, 68.

G. Richter (1963) Z. Naturforschung 18b, 1085.

H.G. Schweiger and S. Berger (1964) Protoplasma 64, 1.

H.G. Schweiger and H.J. Bremer (1960) Exptl. Cell Res. 20, 617.

H.G. Schweiger and H.J. Bremer (1961) Biochim. Biophys. Acta 51, 50.

E. Schweiger, H.G. Wallraff and H.G. Schweiger (1964) Science 146, 658.

D. Shephard (1965a) Biochim. Biophys. Acta 108, 635.

D. Shephard (1965b) Exptl. Cell Res. 37, 93.

T. Spencer and H. Harris (1964) Biochem. J. 91, 282.

S. Sussman (1965) Brookhaven Symposia in Biology, June 7-9.

Triplett, E.L., A. Steens-Lievens and E. Baltus (1965) Exptl. Cell Res. 38, 366.

T. Vanden Driessche (1967) Nach. Akad. Wissens. Göttingen 10, 108.

T. Vanden Driessche and S. Bonotto (1969) Biochim. Biophys. Acta 179, 58.

K.Zetsche (1965) Planta 64, 119.

SUBJECT INDEX

A

Acetabularia
  calyculus, 179
  (Polyphysa) cliftonii, 135-143
  crenulata, 10, 74, 88, 97, 178, 216, 221
  mediterranea, 3, 10, 17-34, 35, 46, 61,
    74, 77, 87, 88, 96, 98, 111, 119,
    134, 145, 177-180, 186-188, 195,
    196, 213, 216, 221, 239, 240, 255,
    256, 275
Acids, 180, 183, 190
Actidione, *see* cycloheximide
Actinomycin, 18, 90, 91, 103, 106, 127,
    182, 183, 236, 239, 243, 244, 254,
    258, 277, 281, 285
  staining with ^{3}H-actinomycin, 277
  micro-injection of, 284
Adenosinetriphosphate (ATP), 5, 215,
    219, 232
  rhythm of, 215
Allosteric proteins, 213, 221, 227
Amino acids, *see also* names of specific
    amino acids, 180, 183, 184, 239,
    240, 241, 243, 248, 251, 253
    274, 285
  composition of lamellar proteins, 251
Amphibian eggs, 284
Amylose, 221
Anyloplasts, 198
Amytal, inhibitor of mitochondria, 200
Anacystis nidulans, DNA content, 46
Antibiotics, *see also* names of specific
    antibiotics, 37, 38, 244, 274
Anthoceros, mitochondria in, 152
Apico-basal gradient

  of long, and of globular chloro-
    plasts, 112, 114
  of "morphogenetic substances", 46, 284
  of m-RNA, 94, 95, 281
  of nuclear substances, 115
  of nucleic acids, 224
  of RNA, 18
  of UDPG - pyrophosphorylose, 92, 94,
    106, 107, 109, 284
Aplysia, 226
ATP, *see* adenosine triphosphate
Autoradiography, 18, 75

B

Bacteria
  contamination by, 38, 39, 200, 204
    205, 239, 242, 243, 278
  DNA of, 40, 46, 64
  protein synthesis in, 243
  RNA of, 39
Blue-green algae, DNA content, 46

C

Calvin cycle, 195, 202, 221
  intermediates of the, 202
Cap
  formation, 4, 17, 19, 24-26, 37, 61,
    64, 66, 87, 89-92, 95, 131, 146,
    177, 214, 255-257, 259, 261, 266,
    273, 276, 278, 280
  inhibitory effects of the nucleus upon
    cap formation, 91
  growth, effect of radiation, 262, 263

293